The
Early Sprouts
Cookbook

Another Redleaf Book by Karrie Kalich

*Early Sprouts: Cultivating Healthy Food Choices in Young Children*
— Karrie Kalich, Dottie Bauer, and Deirdre McPartlin

# *the* Early Sprouts Cookbook

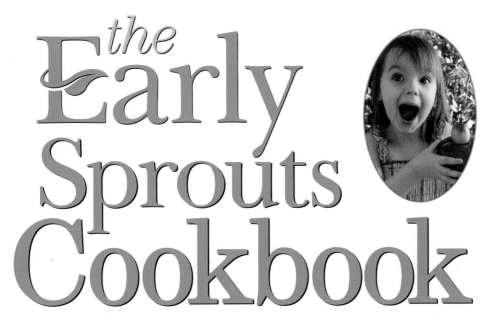

Karrie Kalich ❧ Lynn Arnold ❧ Carole Russell

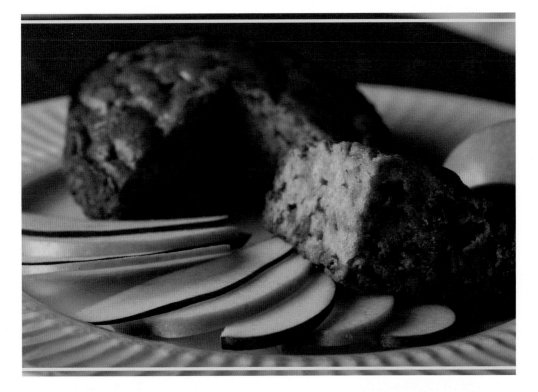

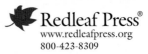

Redleaf Press®
www.redleafpress.org
800-423-8309

Published by Redleaf Press
10 Yorkton Court
St. Paul, MN 55117
www.redleafpress.org

First edition 2012
Cover design by Jim Handrigan
Cover photograph by William Wrobel. Cover inset photograph by
  iStockphoto.com/Karen Squires
Illustrations by Chris Wold Dyrud
Interior typeset in Adobe Caslon and Geometric 415 and designed by
  Jim Handrigan
Interior photos by William Wrobel except for photographs on pages 82, 101,
  133, 141, and 144 by Jim Handrigan
Printed in the United States of America
18 17 16 15 14 13 12 11      1 2 3 4 5 6 7 8

Library of Congress Cataloging-in-Publication Data

Kalich, Karrie.
   The early sprouts cookbook / Karrie Kalich, Lynn Arnold, and
   Carole Russell. — 1st ed.
      p. cm.
   Includes bibliographical references and index.
   ISBN 978-1-60554-042-9 (alk. paper)
   1. Preschool children—Nutrition.  2. Cooking.  3. Food preferences.
   4. Cookbooks.    I. Arnold, Lynn.  II. Russell, Carole.  III. Title.
TX361.C5K352 2011
649'.3—dc23
                                        2011014234

Printed on acid-free paper

TO OUR CHILDREN:

CHRIS, DAN, LEAH, GRADY, AND COOPER

———⌇———

IN MEMORY OF

SUZAN SCHAFER-MEISZNER

# Contents

# Acknowledgments

We would like to thank the individuals who have contributed to the creation of this book in meaningful ways:

The children, staff, and administrators at the Keene State College Child Development Center, Keene Head Start, and the Children's Learning Center at Dartmouth-Hitchcock in Keene who assisted in testing all of the recipes and providing insightful feedback.

Jeanny Aldrich (food stylist) and William Wrobel (photographer) for their creativity and professionalism.

The Keene State College Health Science Nutrition students who contributed time and energy to testing the recipes with the preschool children: Jamie Buccheri, Lindsey Austin, and Nicole Ferri. Also thank you to Leah Arnold, who helped to document the process.

Deirdre McPartlin, Ellen Edge, Dottie Bauer, and Suzan Schafer-Meiszner for their support, mentorship, and willingness to assist in furthering the Early Sprouts goals and vision.

Our spouses—Kris Arnold, David Payson, and Tim Sampson—who provided us with time to work on the book and enthusiastically tasted each recipe.

The generous funders who believe in and support our work:

- Advocates for Healthy Youth

- Cheshire Health Foundation

- CMH Foundation

- Gemini Fund of the New Hampshire Charitable Foundation

- Hannaford supermarkets

- HNH*foundation*

- Monadnock Challenge Fund of the New Hampshire Charitable Foundation

- Environmental Education Fund of the New Hampshire Charitable Foundation

- Our families and friends

Finally, to the people at Redleaf Press for making this such an enjoyable experience.

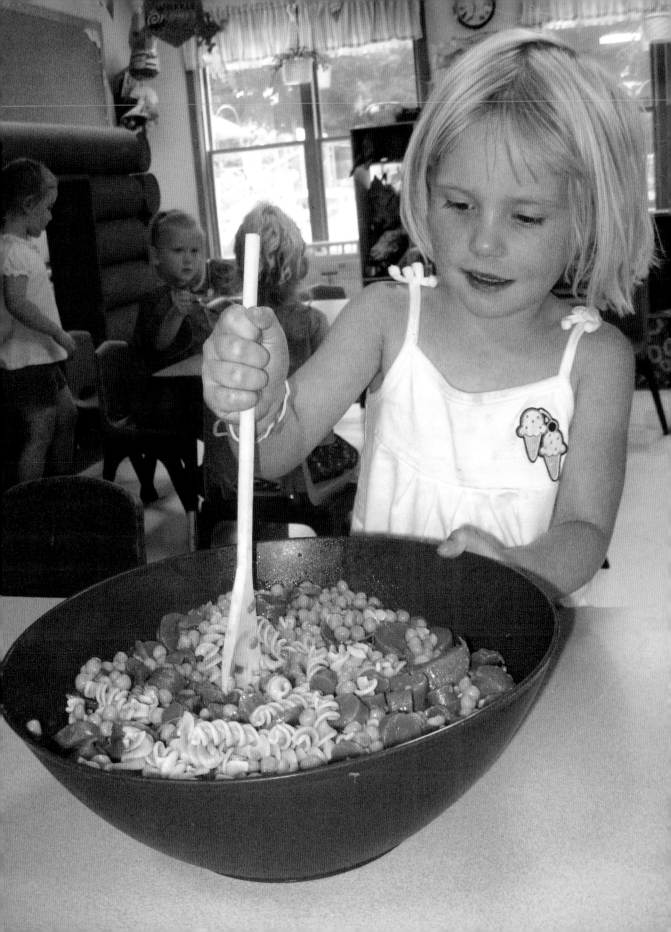

# ONE

—〰—

# The Importance of Nutrition in the Early Childhood Years

The preschool years are an exciting time for children and their caregivers—so much growth and development take place! Good nutrition is crucial to preschoolers' health, but many challenges are involved in helping young children develop healthy eating habits. Preschool-age children are starting to become aware of and manipulated by advertising. Their parents may be swayed by marketing ploys as well. Children may be influenced by what they see their friends and older siblings eating. What we call kids' foods in this book are colorful, appealing, interactive, and relentlessly marketed to young children, often by some of their favorite TV characters. Unfortunately, these foods are almost always high in sugar, fat, and sodium and low in nutritional value. The advertising dollars spent on marketing sweetened cereals, soft drinks, salty snacks, and fast food dramatically exceed those used to promote vegetables and nutrition education programs (Gallo 1999). The preschool years are also notorious for being the time when many children who ate (or at least tried) everything offered to them in infancy and toddlerhood suddenly become very picky eaters, rejecting the healthy foods they used to eat willingly.

Parents often find themselves using coercion—"No dessert until your broccoli is gone!"—or deception—hiding puréed vegetables in the brownies—to get their children to eat healthy foods. The Early Sprouts approach is different: its goal is to help children (and their families) choose to eat healthy foods such as fruits, vegetables, and whole grains. Instilling healthy eating behaviors in preschool children through a positive approach assists in the development of positive lifelong habits. These healthy habits decrease the risk of obesity and other related chronic diseases while contributing to children's growth and development. It may be tempting to hold families responsible for establishing healthy eating patterns in young children, but doing so isn't realistic. When one considers that preschool-age children may be eating up to two meals and one or two snacks per day in a child care setting or preschool, it becomes clear that educators must share this responsibility with parents, particularly if the program provides meals as well as snacks.

## THE OBESITY EPIDEMIC

The increase in the percentage of the United States population who are either overweight or obese is one of the fastest-growing public health concerns. Some of the most dramatic increases in the rates of overweight and obesity have been observed in preschool-age children. In this age group, the prevalence of obesity has more than doubled in the past thirty years (Hessert 2005). This problem has reached epidemic proportions, with nearly 25 percent of children ages two to five considered to be overweight and more than 12 percent categorized as obese (Ogden, Carroll, and Flegal 2008). Children who are obese or overweight carry a high risk of remaining overweight in adulthood, increasing their risk for developing chronic diseases later in life. Even more alarming is the increase in adult diseases and conditions, such as type 2 diabetes and early signs of heart disease, that are now being observed in children and adolescents. As awareness of and concern for overweight and obesity in young children have increased, educators and public health professionals have recognized the importance of addressing the issue in the early years. This is particularly important for prevention.

Obesity in children has many causes. The major factors contributing to childhood obesity fall into two broad categories: (1) too little physical activity and (2) poor dietary habits. Children are too sedentary and consume too many processed foods that are low in nutritional value and high in added sugars, unhealthy fats, sodium, and calories. At the same time, children do not eat enough of the foods that promote health and contribute to maintenance of a healthy body weight: fruits and vegetables, whole grains, lean protein, low-fat dairy products and other calcium-rich foods, and healthy oils.

## HEALTHY EATING FOR PRESCHOOL CHILDREN

The United States Department of Agriculture (USDA), creator of the USDA Food Guidance System, publishes guidelines for a healthy diet on its website at www.choosemyplate.gov. MyPlate, the icon that replaced the Food

Guide Pyramid in 2011, reflects current research on the importance of various nutrients and foods. The graphic helps consumers choose a healthy diet by illustrating the relative importance of different food groups at every meal, with an emphasis on consuming fruits and vegetables. According to MyPlate, one-half of the plate at every meal should be filled with choices from these groups. The USDA recommendations differ according to age, activity level, and gender. The website offers nutrition information for specific audiences, including preschool-aged children. One of the features of the website allows users to customize dietary recommendations for young children based on age, sex, and activity level. In addition, parents and caregivers can find information to help plan menus, as well as resources for additional nutrition information. The website also features tips for becoming a healthy role model, suggestions for feeding picky eaters, and ideas for including children in cooking activities.

MyPlate recommends that daily intake should include choices from these five food groups:

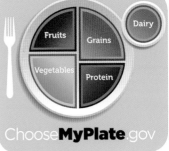

1. Grains, half of which should be whole grains

2. Vegetables

3. Fruits

4. Dairy products

5. Protein foods, such as lean meats, poultry, fish, dry beans, legumes, and nuts.

Selecting a variety of these foods on a weekly basis contributes to a healthy diet. For example, dark green leafy vegetables and orange vegetables supply different important nutrients. Be sure to include both in your weekly menus. Fresh fruits are preferred, and fruit juices should be limited or eliminated because of their concentrated sugar content. It is also important to limit extras, such as sugary foods and snacks, and to include healthy oils while decreasing consumption of *trans* and saturated fats. The USDA recommends physical activity as an important component of healthy diet. The recommendation for children is a minimum of sixty minutes of physical activity on most or all days each week (United States Department of Agriculture and United States Department of Health Human Services 2010).

Adults need to remember that children's dietary needs are different from those of adults, both in portion size and nutritional composition. For example, preschool-age children should consume 1½–2 cups of vegetables and 1–1½ cups of fruit daily. MyPlate also recommends that young children consume two servings of low-fat or fat-free dairy products and 3–5 ounces of protein foods each day. Finally, it recommends that young children consume 4–5 ounces of grains (bread, cereal, rice, or pasta) every day, half of these

**Table 1**     SERVING AMOUNTS AND SIZES
### Recommended by the USDA for Preschoolers
### Based on a 1,400 Calorie Diet (www.choosemyplate.gov/preschoolers/)

| FOOD GROUP | DAILY SERVINGS | SERVING SIZES |
|---|---|---|
| Grains Group | 5 oz.<br>(half should be<br>whole grains) | 1 oz. is equal to<br>1 slice bread<br>1 cup ready-to-eat cereal<br>½ cup cooked cereal, rice, or pasta |
| Vegetable Group | 1½ cups | cooked or raw vegetables<br>raw leafy vegetables (1 cup of raw leafy<br>   vegetables = ½ cup vegetables)<br>vegetable juice |
| Fruit Group | 1½ cups | medium apple, banana, orange, pear<br>chopped, cooked, or canned fruit<br>100% fruit juice (no more than 6 oz./day) |
| Dairy Group (preferably fat-free or low-fat) | 2 cups | milk or yogurt<br>natural cheese (such as cheddar;<br>   1½ oz. = 1 cup of milk)<br>processed cheeses (such as American;<br>   2 oz. = 1 cup of milk) |
| Protein Foods Group | 4 oz. | lean meat, poultry, or fish<br>The following count as 1 ounce of meat:<br>¼ cup of cooked dry beans<br>2 tbsp hummus<br>1 egg<br>1 tbsp peanut butter<br>½ oz. nuts or seeds |

being whole grains. As with adults, preschoolers' needs vary according to their age and activity level. Table 1 summarizes the USDA recommendations for a typical four-year-old who gets the recommended sixty minutes of physical activity each day.

Dietitians and public health officials recommend a diet rich in fruits, vegetables, and whole grains, partly because these foods help people achieve and maintain healthy body weight. These nutrient-dense foods are important in young children's diets because of their high vitamin and mineral content, which supports healthy physical growth and development. *Nutrient density* means that a serving provides a significant amount of important nutrients without contributing too many calories to total daily intake. Fruits, vegetables, and whole grains are rich in fiber, which contains no absorbable calories but contributes to a feeling of fullness or satiety. Fruits and vegetables also contain water, which makes one feel full without adding calories. Total calories and activity level are also related. A person who eats more calories than are used in activities of daily living and daily exercise gains weight. A person who eats fewer calories than are used loses weight.

Fruits and vegetables are especially important to eat because of their role as a natural source of essential vitamins, minerals, and phytochemicals, such as beta-carotene. In fact, consuming a diet rich in fruits and vegetables helps to protect against several chronic diseases. Compared to people who consume a minimal amount of fruits and vegetables, those who eat generous amounts have decreased risks of cardiovascular diseases, strokes, and certain cancers.

A large majority of children from two to five years of age in the United States don't meet most of the dietary guidelines set forth by the USDA. These children fall short of the recommended number of vegetable servings (especially dark leafy greens and orange vegetables), whole grains, meat and beans, and vegetable and fish oils. On the other hand, children in this age group eat more than a moderate amount of saturated fats, sodium, and extra calories from added sugars and saturated and *trans* fats (Fungwe et al. 2009). The American Heart Association recommends that children from four to eight years of age consume no more than three teaspoons of added sugars per day (Johnson et al. 2009), but the average intake of added sugars in this age group is twenty-one teaspoons per day (National Cancer Institute 2010).

## VEGETABLES

To maximize their nutritional benefit, a wide variety of vegetables should be consumed. Vegetables of different colors provide different nutrients, and the frequently offered advice to "eat a rainbow" is an effective way to teach children to incorporate a variety of vegetables (and fruit) into their diet. Carrots, sweet potatoes, and winter squashes are rich sources of beta-carotene. Tomatoes and red peppers are excellent sources of vitamin C. Leafy greens, such as Swiss chard and spinach, and other green veggies, such as broccoli and green beans, contain many vitamins and minerals, including calcium and iron. White vegetables, such as parsnips and cauliflower, have significant health benefits as well. All vegetables are a good source of dietary fiber. Canned vegetables lose some of their vitamin content during processing and tend to be high in sodium. Nevertheless, canned vegetables without added salt retain some of their phytochemicals and can be part of a healthy diet. Overall, fresh, frozen, or no-salt-added canned vegetables are recommended.

### THE IMPORTANCE OF WHOLE FOODS

The closer a food is to being whole (in its original, unprocessed state), the greater its nutritional value. When foods or their ingredients are processed or refined, nutrients are likely to be lost and unhealthy ingredients—sugar, sodium, and saturated fat—are likely to be added. For example, an apple contains vitamins, minerals, fiber, and phytochemicals that contribute to health. When the fruit is processed into applesauce, the peel is removed, taking away much of the fiber and some of the vitamins. Turn the apple into juice, and a further loss of fiber and vitamins occurs while the concentration of sugar and number of calories increase. At the other end of the wholeness scale from the original apple, you'll find the very popular chewy fruit snacks, which are made from apple juice with added sugar, corn syrup, cornstarch, and artificial colors. The nutrient-dense apple has become a calorie-dense, highly processed product that is much closer to candy than fruit. A good rule of thumb when considering food choices is to try to picture the food growing on a tree or in a garden. If it's hard to imagine that toaster pastry hanging from a branch, then the bowl of fresh blueberries is going to be a better choice.

## PHYTOCHEMICALS AND ANTIOXIDANTS

In addition to nutrients like vitamins and minerals, many foods derived from plants contain antioxidants and phytochemicals. These substances are not necessary for our survival the way vitamins and minerals are, but they are thought to contribute greatly to preventing disease and improving health. Phytochemicals are compounds that are found in plants (*phyto* means "plant" in Greek) and protect the plant from insects, microorganisms, and sunlight. In humans, phytochemicals are thought to help prevent chronic diseases. Many phytochemicals are associated with plant pigments, which is one of the reasons people are urged to consume a variety of colored fruits and vegetables. Scientists have identified several thousand different phytochemicals and expect to find more. Some phytochemicals are antioxidants. Antioxidants are compounds that neutralize free radicals, which are charged particles that our bodies produce as a result of normal metabolism. Free radicals are also produced by pollution and exposure to sunlight. If they are not neutralized by antioxidants, they can cause damage to our cells, leading to diseases like cancer and cardiovascular disease. Some vitamins and minerals also function as antioxidants—vitamin C and selenium are good examples. It's also believed that the way phytochemicals interact with each other and with other nutrients in food increases the positive effects they have on our health. There are too many phytochemicals to make it practical to ingest them in supplement form, so the best way to get these important compounds is by eating a wide variety of plant-based foods.

## FRUIT

It is important to eat a wide variety of fruits. While many vegetables are naturally somewhat bitter in flavor, fruits taste sweeter because of their fruit sugar or fructose. Young children often enjoy eating fruit more than vegetables. As with vegetables, eating different colored fruits each day contributes to a healthy diet, because different fruits provide different nutrients. For example, bananas are a rich source of potassium, while citrus fruits are an excellent source of vitamin C. Deeply colored berries and cherries contain antioxidants and other phytochemicals. Whole or cut-up fruit is more nutritious than fruit juice. Whole fruits are richer in dietary fiber and lower in total sugar per serving than juice. When possible, choose fresh or frozen (without added sugar) fruit over canned fruit. Canned fruit without added sugar and packed in its own juice can also contribute to a healthy diet.

Here are some ways to increase fruit and vegetable intake (for all ages):

- Add blueberries, bananas, or dried fruit to hot or cold breakfast cereals.

- Make a fruit smoothie for breakfast or for a refreshing snack.

- Add berries, dried fruit, or chopped apples to muffin and pancake batters.

- Top French toast with apple sauce.

- Stuff an omelet with sautéed vegetables, such as onions, peppers, mushrooms, and zucchini.

- Top sandwiches with extra veggies, such as lettuce, peppers, tomato slices, grated carrots, or raw, shredded beets.

- Keep a bowl of sliced fruits, such as melons or pineapple, in the fridge for quick and easy snacking.

- Add chopped vegetables to pasta sauces or use them as pizza toppings.

- Grill vegetables, such as eggplant, summer squash, zucchini, peppers, and asparagus, for a tasty and healthy summer cookout side dish.

- Top frozen yogurt with fresh berries.

- Pack a piece of fresh fruit or a baggie of sliced vegetables for a snack any time of the day.

- Have a vegetarian main dish once or twice a week.

## WHOLE GRAINS

In addition to fruits and vegetables, whole grains are important for maintaining health. Whole grains include brown rice, whole grain pasta, barley, spelt, oatmeal, whole wheat flour (red wheat), cornmeal, white whole wheat flour, whole wheat couscous, whole grain cereals, quinoa, millet, and bulgur. As preschoolers, children can learn to enjoy whole grains. These habits and taste preferences will help them sustain healthy eating patterns as they mature and become adults. The advice to "make half your grains whole" is the minimum recommendation. It's desirable to make even more of your grain choices whole grains.

Whole grains are a more complete source of nutrition than their processed cousins. Whole grains contain more vitamins, minerals, and dietary fiber than processed grains, such as bleached or unbleached all-purpose flour, white rice, and white pasta. In processed grains, the bran and germ have been removed by polishing. These nutritional components are then sold separately in forms like wheat germ and bran cereal. Although some of the vitamins and minerals that have been removed by refining grains are added back when flour is enriched, the majority of these important nutrients are lost when grains are processed. An easy way to add whole grains to your diet is to substitute them for the processed grains you are already eating. People who have adjusted to a change to whole grains usually report that they enjoy the nutty flavor and chewier texture of whole grains and find the refined grain foods they used to eat bland and lacking in flavor.

### HOW CAN WHITE FLOUR BE WHOLE WHEAT?

White whole wheat flour is made from a strain of wheat with less pigmentation in the bran than traditional whole wheat flour has. Because it is the pigments that give whole wheat flour the stronger flavor that some people object to, foods made with white whole wheat have a milder flavor as well as a lighter color. Baked goods also have a lighter texture when made with white whole wheat flour compared to those made with traditional whole wheat flour. White whole wheat flour is still made from the whole grain and contains all of the nutrition associated with whole wheat flour, making it a great choice for baking.

Here are some ways to substitute whole grains for processed grains in children's diets:

- Use brown rice, quinoa, spelt, or wheat berries instead of white rice.

- Choose a whole grain cereal, such as oatmeal, over a processed grain cereal.

- Select stone-ground whole wheat bread over white bread.

Many health benefits are associated with consuming dietary fiber from fruits, vegetables, legumes, and whole grains. For example, dietary fiber

- improves bowel function and prevents constipation
- reduces the risk of developing hemorrhoids and diverticula (small pouches in the lining of the colon)
- contributes to the maintenance of healthy weight
- reduces the risk of obesity by making us feel full without a lot of calories
- assists with regulating blood sugar levels
- helps manage blood cholesterol levels
- reduces the risk of colon cancer

Look for dietary fiber on food labels. Try to choose products with 2–5 grams of fiber per serving. The American Heart Association's recommendation for fiber intake for preschoolers is 19 grams per day for three-year-olds and 25 grams for four- and five-year-olds. It's better to choose foods that are naturally rich in fiber than foods that have fiber added to them. (See page 63 for more suggestions for increasing fiber intake.)

- Replace ⅓ to ½ of the all-purpose flour in your favorite recipes with whole wheat flour.

- Exchange 100 percent of the all-purpose flour in a favorite recipe with white whole wheat flour or whole wheat pastry flour.

- Substitute whole grain pastas for white pastas.

- Use barley in soups instead of noodles.

## DAIRY

Dairy-based foods are a rich source of calcium and vitamin D. Both of these nutrients are important for bone growth and development. Calcium is also important to contract muscles, transmit nerve impulses, and assist with proper blood clotting. In addition, it may play a role in maintaining healthy weight. Many dairy products, such as whole milk, whole milk yogurt, cream, half-and-half, sour cream, cream cheese, and ice cream, are high sources of saturated fat. This type of fat is a key contributor to heart disease. For that reason, low-fat or fat-free calcium-rich foods are key components in a healthy diet. While children under the age of two should be given only whole-milk dairy products, once past that age they should consume low- or nonfat dairy foods. Encouraging children to establish the habit of consuming low- or nonfat milk and yogurt at an early age will set them up with a lifelong healthy habit. Since every cell in our bodies needs calcium, consuming dairy or a calcium-fortified dairy substitute on a daily basis is important. Fat-free and 1 percent milk are good choices, as are low-fat cheeses and low-fat or fat-free yogurts.

Numerous dairy-free alternatives are available for those who are lactose intolerant or have a dairy allergy. Select fortified soy-, rice-, or nut-based products. The quality and variety of these products are constantly improving. Select a product that is fortified with calcium and vitamin D but not loaded with added sugars. Many people who are lactose intolerant are able to eat yogurt or cheese because these foods contain only small amounts of lactose; lactose-free milks are also available. Nondairy foods can provide calcium—for example, calcium-fortified orange juice and tofu, canned salmon, and vegetables like bok choy, kale, and broccoli.

Before buying flavored yogurt, check its sugar content. Many of the fruited yogurts currently available, including those that are marketed specifically to young children, contain over 2 tablespoons of sugar per 6-ounce serving. This is more than twice the recommended limit of 3 teaspoons of sugar per day. Sugar contains empty calories, meaning it is high in calories but contains no vitamins or minerals. If eating plain yogurt is less enjoyable, add fresh fruit to it or combine plain yogurt with a favorite fruited yogurt.

Vitamin D, the sunshine vitamin, is as important as calcium for bone growth and development. In fact, without vitamin D, our bones cannot absorb calcium. Exposing the hands, arms, and face to the sun provides vitamin D. In northern climates during the winter months, a negligible amount of vitamin D is available from sunlight, so it must be consumed through food or supplements. Common foods, including fat-free or low-fat milk and milk products, fortified breakfast cereals, and eggs, can help to meet our vitamin D needs.

**HOW MUCH SUGAR IS IN A GRAM?**

When you read a Nutrition Facts label, the sugar content is always measured in grams. What does that mean to those of us who are used to measuring ingredients in terms of teaspoons and tablespoons? A teaspoon of sugar contains approximately 4 grams of sugar; a tablespoon has about 12 grams. So if the label says a cup of children's cereal has 12 grams of sugar, that means there is a full tablespoon of sugar in that one-cup serving. And that 12-ounce can of cola, with 39 grams of sugar, contains 9¾ teaspoons of sugar!

## LEAN PROTEIN

Foods that are healthy sources of protein include lean meats, fish, dried beans, tofu, nuts, seeds, and eggs. Protein is found throughout the body in tissues such as bone, skin, and muscle. Protein is also an important component of the many enzymes and hormones that regulate the body's physiological processes. Although the rate at which a child grows during the preschool years is slower than during infancy and toddlerhood, every child still needs adequate amounts of protein to continue building a healthy body.

Some meats, although rich in protein, also contain significant amounts of saturated fat, which can contribute to the risk of heart disease. Choosing lean cuts of meat or sources that are lower in saturated fat, such as chicken or turkey breast, is important. Fish is a healthy choice for protein because it contains healthy omega 3 fatty acids and little saturated fat. Women of child-bearing age and young children should avoid fish that are likely to have high levels of mercury, especially shark, swordfish, tilefish, and king mackerel. Canned light tuna is lower in mercury than canned white (albacore) tuna; salmon, haddock, tilapia, and catfish are all good choices. Eggs are also a good sources of protein. Studies have found that the dietary cholesterol contained in eggs does not contribute to increased blood cholesterol levels (the saturated fat in meat is more likely to do that). Plant proteins, such as beans and nuts, are very low in saturated fat and contain healthy oils as well as fiber (which is not found in animal protein). Beans are also very economical—they are the least expensive protein food you can buy, besides being one of the healthiest.

## HEALTHY FATS

During the 1990s, dietary advice often called for keeping consumption of all fats as low as possible. Since then, we have learned that there are different types of fats and that not all of them are unhealthy. Research has shown that saturated and *trans* fats contribute to the development of heart disease and some cancers. Yet the liquid oils found in many plant-based foods and fish actually contribute to heart health and overall wellness. Oils are very calorie-dense, and they contain more than twice as many calories per gram as proteins and carbohydrates. While we don't need large amounts of them, some plant oils in the diet every day are desirable. Examples of good choices include olive, canola, and safflower oils, nuts, and avocados. Plant oils contain the fatty acids that are essential (in other words, they must be consumed because our bodies cannot make them). The concentrated dose of calories that comes with oils may be desirable for preschoolers, who need more calories than their small stomachs may be able to hold. Finally, some fats are needed so children can absorb the fat-soluble vitamins found in food: vitamins A, D, E, and K. The MyPlate recommendation for oils for a preschooler is 3–4 teaspoons per day.

## WATER

Using water to quench thirst is another good health habit to establish during the preschool years. Many parents and caregivers offer young children liberal quantities of fruit juice, believing that it is a healthy choice. Children drink it quite happily because it is sweet. Nevertheless, the high level of sugars in even 100 percent fruit juice makes it a much less desirable choice than eating a whole fruit. Some juices, such as apple or white grape juice, are virtually sugar water, offering very little nutritional value. Fruit-flavored drinks and soda are even worse, containing nothing but empty calories. Sports drinks are only justified when children are engaged in vigorous physical activity for long stretches of time. We recommend that you do not make juice a component of children's regular diet. If you're going to offer juice to children, limit it to no more than 6 ounces per day, and offer a type of juice that is more nutritionally valuable, such as 100 percent orange or purple grape juice. Better yet, give children a piece of fresh fruit and a cup of water!

## READING NUTRITION LABELS

Becoming a savvy food label reader is crucial to good nutrition. It's important to understand what information can be found in both the Nutrition Facts panel and the ingredients list on a food package. This information can be used in planning a healthy diet.

Be sure to pay attention to the serving size and number of servings per container listed on the Nutrition Facts label. It's not unusual for people to eat more than the listed serving size of a particular food. If you eat twice as much as the serving listed on the label, then all of the numbers on the label need to be doubled—twice as many calories, twice as many grams of sugar, fiber, and so on. Serving sizes for preschoolers will often be smaller than the serving size given on the Nutrition Facts label. In that case, the number of calories and grams of nutrients will be some fraction of what the label states.

The % Daily Value (DV) on the Nutrition Facts label is based on a 2,000 calorie diet, which is a typical adult intake. Preschool-age children are likely to have a daily intake of 1,200–1,600 calories. However, it's still possible to use the % DV on the label as a way of gauging adequate or excessive intake of some nutrients. If a food contains less than 5 percent of the DV of a particular nutrient, it is considered to be low in that nutrient. If it contains more than 20 percent, it is high in that nutrient, regardless of how many calories are required by a person on a daily basis.

The nutrients listed in the first part of the Nutrition Facts label are the ones to limit: saturated and *trans* fats, cholesterol, and sodium. Nutrients that many people need to get more of are found further down on the label: potassium, fiber, vitamins A and C, calcium, and iron.

---

**Fig. 1**               **NUTRITION FACTS**

# Nutrition Facts

Serving size  (1 cup)  (243g)
Servings per container about (2)

Check the serving size and number of servings per container to be sure the nutrition information applies to the portion you're eating.

**Amount Per Serving**

**Calories**   150   Calories from fat   **25**

**% Daily Value***

| | |
|---|---|
| **Total Fat**   1g | **2%** |
| Saturated Fat   .5g | (**3%**) |
| **Cholesterol**   10mg | **3%** |
| **Sodium**   730mg | (**30%**) |
| **Total Carbohydrates**   25g | **8%** |
| Dietary Fiber   4g | **16%** |
| Sugars   4g | |
| **Protein**   9g | |

Less than 5% indicates this food is low in saturated fat.

More than 20% indicates this food is high in sodium.

Eat less of these.

Eat more of these.

| | | | |
|---|---|---|---|
| Vitamin A | **15%** | Vitamin C | **0%** |
| Calcium | **2%** | Iron | **6%** |

*Percent Daily Values are based on a 2,000 calorie diet.

Sometimes you may find that a food label claims that the product is an "excellent source" or "good source" of a nutrient such as calcium, fiber, or a particular vitamin. Foods that are an "excellent source" of a nutrient must provide 20 percent or more of the Recommended Daily Value, based on USDA guidelines. Foods that are a "good source" of a nutrient must provide 10–19 percent of the USDA Recommended Daily Value.

The ingredients list contains all of the ingredients in that food, listed in order by weight. The product contains more of the first ingredient than any of the other ingredients. The longer the ingredients list, the more likely the food is to be highly processed and therefore less healthy, especially if many of the ingredients sound unfamiliar.

How the product looks or what the front of the package says can be deceiving. You usually need to look at the ingredients list in order to tell if the food is a whole grain product. Bread that is brown in color may be whole grain bread, or it may be made from white flour that has been colored with molasses. If the front of the package reads "made with whole grains," that means the product is at least partly made with whole grains. If the ingredients list reads "enriched wheat flour," this tells you that the food is not 100 percent whole grain. Look for words such as "100% whole grain," "whole wheat flour," and "whole grain rye flour" to determine if the product is a whole grain food.

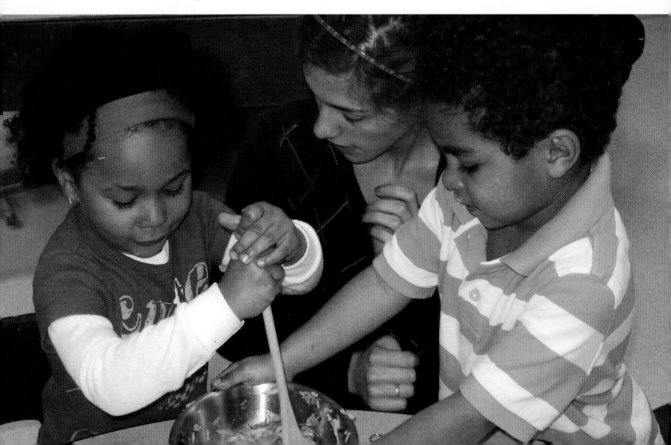

You also need to read the ingredients list carefully to determine the food's sugar content. There are many different words signifying sugar that can appear on labels, such as

- sugar
- high fructose corn syrup
- corn syrup or corn syrup solids
- corn sweetener
- evaporated cane juice
- honey
- molasses
- dextrin

- dextrose
- maltodextrin
- malt syrup
- maltose
- rice syrup
- fruit juice concentrate
- invert sugar

Often more than one of these appears in an ingredients list. Some foods, particularly milk and fruit, contain naturally occurring sugars. The number of grams of sugars found on the Nutrition Facts label includes these natural sugars as well as added sugars. Telling where the sugar comes from can be difficult, so looking at the ingredients list is important: if one of the sugar words is near the beginning of the list or there is more than one sugar word, the food is likely to be high in added sugars.

To find out if a food contains *trans* fats, look at the ingredients. Even though the front of the package may say "*trans* fat free" and the Nutrition Facts label shows 0 grams of *trans* fats, a product may still contain *trans* fats. Labeling laws state that the "*trans* fat free" claim can be made if the food contains less than 0.5 gram *trans* fat per serving. If the ingredients list contains the words "partially hydrogenated" in front of any oils in the list, then the food has *trans* fats in it.

## CHILD AND ADULT CARE FOOD PROGRAM

The Child and Adult Care Food Program (CACFP) is administered on the federal level by the USDA. It provides money for nutritious meals and snacks for children and adults in child care programs, emergency shelters, and after-school programs. Participating child care centers are reimbursed for some or all of the costs of providing up to two meals and one snack, or two snacks and one meal to children. The meals and snacks must, however, meet the requirements outlined by the Food and Nutrition Service/USDA guidelines. Eligibility for the program is determined by children's eligibility for free or reduced-cost meals, based on family income, or the family's participation in other programs, such as Head Start, Temporary Assistance for Needy Families (TANF), and the Supplemental Nutrition Assistance Program (SNAP, formerly known as the food stamp program). Home child care programs may also be eligible for CACFP if they are licensed and have enrollments that meet the guidelines.

The CACFP meal patterns for children are built around food groups, or components, with minimum quantities and serving sizes for each meal or snack (called a *supplement* by CACFP), based on the ages of children being served. The minimum requirements for meal patterns are consistent with the Dietary Guidelines for Americans. There are four component groups: milk, meat or meat alternate, fruits/vegetables, and grains/bread. The number of required components varies. Two components are needed to make a snack, three for a breakfast, and all four components for a lunch (or a supper).

The introduction to each of the recipe chapters outlines the CACFP requirements for that meal for children aged three to five years. The recipes include suggestions for foods that can be served with the recipe dish to meet the CACFP meal or snack requirements. In many cases, the recipe provides a bonus ingredient that does not fulfill the required components but will add extra nutrition to the meal, such as a partial serving of extra fruit, vegetable, whole grains, or dairy. Bear in mind that the requirements outlined by the CACFP are minimum requirements. Children can be served more than these minimal amounts. Older preschoolers, or those who are more active, may need more than the minimum in order to meet their nutrition needs.

In addition to being in line with CACFP requirements, the recipes in this book incorporate the nutrition principles that have been outlined in this chapter and feature healthful ingredients, including

- whole grains, such as whole wheat flour, brown rice, whole grain pasta, rolled oats, bulgur wheat, and stone-ground cornmeal

- fruits and vegetables

- low-fat dairy products, such as skim milk, low-fat or nonfat yogurt, and reduced-fat cheese

- lean proteins, such as beans, eggs, chicken, and turkey

- oils containing healthy fats, such as canola or olive

- reduced amounts of sodium and sugars compared to those in commercially prepared foods

Each recipe is designed to serve eight preschool-age children and two adults; recipes can be doubled for larger classrooms.

—⁓—

# TWO

# THE
# EARLY SPROUTS
# APPROACH

Take a look around a nutritionally purposeful preschool classroom. . . .

In dramatic play, Cathy, a new teacher, is engaging Grady and Kendal in a cooking activity. Cathy is explaining to the children how her salad includes red, yellow, green, orange, and purple vegetables to ensure it gives her body everything it needs. At the science table, Chris and Dan are carefully investigating the seeds gathered from the bell peppers served at the previous day's lunch. Juan is painting at the easel; when asked to describe his painting, he reports, "This is my family at dinnertime. We are eating carrots. They are good for you." Leah and Cooper are working with colorful blocks at the math table and comparing the colors of the blocks to their favorite fruits and vegetables. At circle time, the class discusses their snack and lunch. The teacher reminds the children that they will have the opportunity to help prepare the whole grain vegetable pizza for lunch.

You have just had a glimpse of the day-to-day activities that occur in the nutritionally purposeful preschool classroom. The Early Sprouts approach is committed to a nutritionally purposeful preschool environment. What does this mean? It means that we

- offer healthy foods in a developmentally appropriate manner

- offer foods for celebrations that follow the Early Sprouts guidelines

- provide multiple opportunities for children to try a new food

- understand that people can begin to like a new food if given time, support, and the opportunity to try it

- respect food as something that nourishes us

- involve children in as many aspects of food preparation as possible

- rely on adults to model healthy eating behaviors

- focus on positive food behaviors in children and families

- involve families in food learning experiences

We have had great success with this approach, and believe you will too.

The food choices and habits of young children are strongly influenced by the food available and the messages given about food in their immediate environments. The home and school environments have a significant influence on the dietary habits and choices of young children. The Early Sprouts approach is based on sound nutritional research, principles of behavior change, and a deep knowledge of early childhood curriculum. The approach depends on effective and caring staff and teachers and actively involved families. It provides a nutritionally purposeful environment that assists children in making healthy dietary choices. But most important, it is engaging and developmentally appropriate.

Early Sprouts provides techniques to assist classroom teachers, home child care providers, families, and youth leaders in providing and engaging children with a nutritionally purposeful environment. By sharing the Early Sprouts approach with you, we hope to have a positive impact on the lifelong eating habits and overall health of children.

## THE IMPORTANCE OF STARTING EARLY

Some people question our focus on preschool children, suggesting that we should direct our efforts toward older children who are better able to understand the importance of a healthy diet. Although understanding the value of healthy eating is important, it is even more important that children (and adults) make actual, good dietary choices. Many people with a substantial knowledge of healthy foods are unable to consistently follow a healthy diet. Older children typically must first overcome poor, already established eating habits and then work to establish new, healthier habits. As a nation, we need strategies that help people put their knowledge into action and help them alter their food preferences and behaviors.

In many ways, early childhood is the ideal time to develop healthy eating habits. During this period, young children first establish many of the eating habits they will practice for the rest of their lives. When children are provided with healthy food choices and allowed to determine how much they eat, they can self-regulate their caloric consumption. And they are able to do this without external pressure to eat or not eat (Johnson and Birch 1994). Simply put, a very young child will suddenly stop eating a favorite food when he is full. As children become increasingly aware of the world around them and the external messages about food become more evident, their ability to self-regulate diminishes. Preschool children become more likely to want a food because a friend or family member is eating it. They may want it because they have seen it advertised. They learn to eat because it is mealtime and are less likely to respond to their own internal hunger or satiety. Because of these factors, the preschool years are an appropriate time to teach healthy eating by modeling healthy behaviors and offering opportunities to try healthy foods. It is much easier and more effective to teach healthy behaviors about food than to undo unhealthy ones.

## THE EARLY SPROUTS NUTRITIONAL PHILOSOPHY

To help young children and their families establish healthy dietary behaviors, we based the Early Sprouts approach on an understanding of how young children establish their food preferences. Three major factors contribute to the dietary habits of young children:

1. Innate presence of food neophobia (fear of new things)

2. Increased influence of environmental and social messages about food

3. Approaches used by many well-intentioned adults when offering foods to young children

We have designed the Early Sprouts program to take these factors into account. Early Sprouts provides strategies to shift young children's food preferences in a positive, healthy direction. We address food neophobia, suggest positive ways to apply environmental and social influences to preschoolers, and provide alternative techniques for adults who are trying to encourage children to eat healthily.

Neophobia (fear of new things) has evolutionary roots in the Paleolithic era. Early humans did not necessarily know whether newly encountered food sources would be nourishing or poisonous. Those who were cautious when encountering new foods were more likely to survive. Those who ate everything might become ill or die from ingesting poisonous, contaminated, or rotten food. Even in the face of starvation, survival-oriented humans were reluctant to consume what could have been a lethal food. As a result, our Paleolithic ancestors developed a fear of unknown foods—food neophobia—that has become part of our genetic makeup.

Many children exhibit exaggerated levels of food neophobia, especially when they are exposed to bitter-tasting foods. In premodern times, if a fruit tasted sweet, it was probably safe to eat. If it tasted sour or bitter, it was best avoided. Many vegetables have a slightly bitter flavor, whereas fruits tend to taste sweet. Young children are naturally more accepting of fruits than vegetables. And, of course, they are even more accepting of cookies, candy, soda, ice cream, and other sweetened foods. Most often, children who are not eating enough fruit are not being offered enough fruit. The bitterness of vegetables requires a slightly different and more strategic approach. Repeated, nonthreatening opportunities to taste a new food or vegetable offer children the chance to alter their reactions from rejection to acceptance (Birch and Marlin 1982; Sullivan and Birch 1994).

Starting around three years, children become increasingly aware of environmental and social messages about food. Suddenly they start to request foods by brand name and are increasingly interested in what people around them are eating. Young children will request that a specific food be prepared in a very specific way. The requested foods may just happen to be identical to something regularly packed in a friend's lunch or served at the child's preschool program. For example, three-year-old Mackenzie sits next to her friend Keaton at lunch; they have been eating lunch together for the past two years in their child care center. Shortly after her third birthday, Mackenzie has become very observant of the foods Keaton has in his lunch box. At home she has started to request the same items she admires in Keaton's lunch in her own.

Children also become very in tune with their food environment and the social settings in which foods are offered. They observe that special foods—for example, ice cream, cake, cookies, and chips—are served and eaten during celebrations, such as birthdays, other parties, and holidays. The fun and excitement surrounding these events make cake and ice cream taste even more delicious. Buttered popcorn, soda, and hot dogs are frequently consumed at movies and sporting events, two common recreational pastimes in the lives of many American families. These observations and experiences, coupled with children's natural preferences for sweet and salty foods, result in these foods becoming favorites. In contrast, young children also hear a parent's complaints about the need to eat just a salad or to skip dessert in an effort to manage weight. Children observe other family members' regular refusal to eat broccoli or green beans at a family meal. The child concludes that these healthier foods are less desirable choices.

Foods that are beneficial to health, such as fruits and vegetables, are frequently offered in negative, coercive ways. Sometimes threats and bribes are used, such as "When you finish your green beans, you can have dessert" or "No TV for you tonight unless you clean your plate." Food becomes a reward or a punishment, not a part of healthy living. Sometimes this is what adults heard growing up. Sometimes it is spoken out of frustration about a child's food habits. Nevertheless, these scenarios make vegetables less appealing (Birch and Fisher 1996). Children learn that the adults are in charge of what to eat, when to eat, and how much to eat. This does not lead to the formation of healthy eating habits.

Teachers and family members should be children's most effective role models by offering and enjoying healthy foods in friendly, supportive environments. It is important for early childhood educators to provide as many positive social cues as possible around healthy foods. This can help to counteract social pressures that lead to less healthy choices. Display your enjoyment of fruits and vegetables. Use healthy foods for celebratory events. For example, our Early Sprouts classrooms enjoy the program's Harvest or Butternut Squash Muffins for birthday celebrations. They make Whole Grain Pizza or Broccoli-Cheddar Soup for family events or staff meetings.

It is important to avoid power struggles with young children over food. Effort is better spent in creating positive social environments that support young children's healthy food choices. Positive social environments and nutritious foods foster the development of lifelong, healthy eating habits. For example, apple- or berry-picking with young children can be fun and exciting and prompt children to eat and enjoy the fruits of their labor. Serving raw veggies and low-fat dip as part of a classroom or family picnic can be successful. Both of these examples provide suitable ways for offering healthy foods to young children. Bottom line: early childhood educators and families should maintain control over children's diet not by engaging in a power struggle but instead by monitoring the foods that are introduced, available, and served. When early childhood educators and families focus their efforts, everyone can develop healthy eating habits.

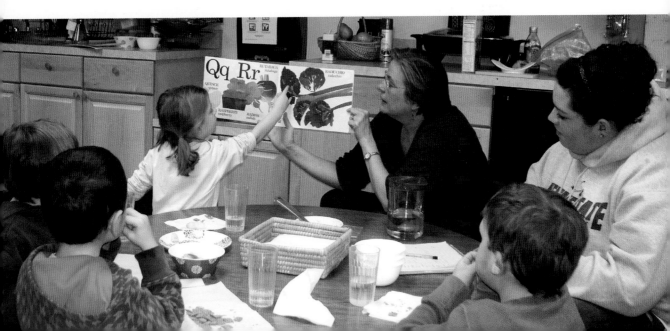

Unfortunately, well-intentioned adults often contribute to the establishment of poor dietary choices, both quantitatively and qualitatively. Coercive approaches or hiding puréed vegetables in a dish may work in the short-term—children may eat vegetables that night. But in the long run, we have not helped them learn to choose these foods and make vegetables a part of daily life. Instilling healthy eating behaviors in preschool children through a positive approach assists in the development of lifelong habits. These healthy habits will decrease the risk of obesity and other chronic diseases.

In the next section of this chapter, we offer specific strategies to influence the dietary choices and behaviors of young children in positive ways:

1. sensory exploration

2. multiple exposures

3. engaging them in food preparation

4. family-style meals

5. intentional language about food

6. providing only healthy choices

7. teacher and families as role models

## SENSORY EXPLORATION

Currently, most Americans are disconnected from their sources of food. Because of this disconnection, it is often necessary to support young children in trying and ultimately enjoying nutritious foods. Young children learn through their senses and movement. Actively involving children in sensory exploration of nutritious foods is an important component of the Early Sprouts approach. By *sensory exploration*, we mean intentionally and actively using all of our senses to interact with and experience a food. The Early Sprouts approach encourages children to use their senses, stimulate their brains, and integrate their various senses through sensory explorations, cooking, and tasting.

Engaging children in sensory exploration provides the opportunity for them to really focus on new food. Posing questions such as "What is inside?" encourages them to make predications, an activity that stimulates scientific exploration. Caregivers or parents can stimulate interest in the food by using nonjudgmental, descriptive words, such as *crunchy, crisp, slippery, sweet*, and *smooth*. Such language helps children understand what they are seeing, hearing, tasting, and smelling. You may decide to sample a green, a yellow, and a purple bean and come up with words to describe all three. Or you may take time to explore the inside of a cucumber or zucchini with young children.

Sensory exploration encourages children to use their senses. With guidance from a caring adult, children can learn to understand and experience a new food in all of its forms. By focusing on its characteristics and qualities, children increase their knowledge and understanding of food as food. This relates to one of the main goals of Early Sprouts, which is to provide children with multiple exposures in order to overcome food neophobia. Ultimately, this increases their preference for and willingness to eat new foods.

## FOOD AS PLAY?

We do not use food as play objects. Some early childhood programs incorporate food items into the art curriculum, such as painting with vegetables or using grains to create collages. In addition to sand and water, classroom sensory tables may feature cornmeal, rice, or birdseed for tactile stimulation. Other early childhood programs never use food as curriculum material. This decision may be based on philosophical grounds—children are hungry, and food should be used for nourishment only—or not using food as play because young children may not be able to distinguish between food to eat and food to play with. Sometimes the decision not to use food as play is based on recognizing that food is scarce in some young children's homes. Some communities place a greater value on food than most Americans. In the Early Sprouts approach, we do not play with vegetables. Instead, we thoughtfully explore, investigate, and taste them.

## PROVIDING MULTIPLE AND REPEAT EXPOSURES

Repeated, nonthreatening opportunities to taste a new food provide children the chance to move from rejection to acceptance and overcome food neophobia (Birch and Marlin 1982; Sullivan and Birch 1994). When incorporating new recipes into your meal or snack menus, remember to provide several exposures to them. Do not assume that because children did not like it the first time, they never will. Kelly was excited to try out her center's new snack menu. After seven years of serving the same snack, Kelly (an adventurous eater) was ready for something new. The first time she served the children Whole Grain Pasta, Parmesan, and Peas, they approached the snack table with extreme caution. Very few of the children even considered tasting the new food. Kelly ate with enthusiasm and shared her genuine fondness for it. The following week, a few more children showed interest in the snack. After three weeks, virtually every child was enjoying the recipe. Today the snack is one of her classroom's favorites! It is important to trust the process and encourage young children to taste and ultimately enjoy new foods.

Be sure to share the reason behind trying new foods several times. It will not take long before children adopt this approach. In Carol's classroom, four-year-old Clay was a natural leader. Clay would always tell children they needed to try a food at least four times. Carol was never really sure where the four came from. But since Clay's *rule* was having a positive impact, she did not interfere too much with his edict. When Clay turned five, he updated the rule, and everyone was encouraged to try a new food at least five times.

## ENGAGING CHILDREN IN FOOD PREPARATION

The recipes in this book were specifically developed to reflect healthy nutritional principles, use affordable ingredients, and be cooked with the participation of young children. They feature simple directions that maximize children's ability to help make the dish.

Involving children in preparing food has many benefits. Through increased exposure to food, children increase their comfort level with new foods, thus decreasing their food neophobia. Helping to prepare a recipe naturally increases children's excitement and curiosity about a food and boosts their likelihood of tasting and liking it. Finally, cooking helps children develop their fine-motor skills and vocabulary. Children in Early Sprouts classrooms have advanced cooking vocabularies. For example, three-year-old Lauren Elise described the day's cooking activity to her mother at pickup time: "First we cracked the egg, and then we chopped the spinach and mixed them together. Next, we measured the dry ingredients, and then we put it all together with a spoon. We baked it and ate it. It was good."

Children are capable of doing real food-prep work. They need the adults responsible for their care and education to take a little time and plan for their participation. Select cooking tools that assure safety and success. For example, children can use table knives with fine serrations and stir with long-handled wooden spoons. They can use graters to shred carrots or cheese and child-sized kitchen scissors to cut ingredients into small pieces. With adult supervision, they can safely operate a blender or food processor.

## FAMILY-STYLE MEALS

As children age, they become increasingly independent. Serving family-style meals is a wonderful way to offer them independence and freedom while supporting them in learning lifelong healthy food habits. For family-style meals to be successful for young children, use tables, plates, serving bowls, and utensils that are child-appropriate. For example, small, lightweight containers allow children to pass food easily from bowls to plates. Be mindful of the serving utensils you provide. Ideally, one to two scoops yields a child-appropriate serving. Water or milk should be offered in a small pitcher so children can carefully pour the beverage into their own cups without spilling. Family-style meals assist children in developing motor skills, positive social relationships, self-esteem, table manners, and independence. From a nutrition perspective, family-style meals offer daily opportunities to develop skills in portion control and healthy food choices. Likewise, family-style meals provide a wonderful opportunity for adults to model healthy food choices, adventurousness around new foods, and good table manners.

Tips:

- Place enough food on the table to meet the minimum CACFP requirements for all children and to feed the adults.

- Adults should always join children at the table and consume the same foods and beverages.

- Be sure always to use small serving containers. These assist children in serving themselves and minimize waste if children accidently spill. A small container also minimizes waste when food needs to be discarded because of coughs or sneezes directly on the food.

## USING INTENTIONAL LANGUAGE ABOUT FOOD

The way we use language influences how we think and feel. In carefully selecting the language we use about food, we can guide children in being more open minded and accepting of foods. Choosing descriptive phrases is very important. The Early Sprouts program is intentional in the language it uses. A key phrase in our approach is "I do not like it yet." This phrase serves as the basis of many of our Early Sprouts goals. For example, when a young child tries a food and responds with "I do not like this" or "This is yucky," we are quick to respond with the phrase "You do not like it yet?" or "You might like it the next time you try it." This terminology lets the child know that we understand she does not like the food. It also plants the idea that she may like it the next time she tries it. Sharing this terminology with families is important. Asking them to respond to their child using similar phrasing has two major benefits: (1) it provides a consistent message about foods that are not liked initially, and (2) it serves as a constant reminder (to both parent and child) to offer a food repeatedly as her preferences change. Children exposed to the Early Sprouts approach begin to use this language as well. Hana, a five-year-old, used this language in describing her thoughts about the Early Sprouts veggie burgers to her teacher. "At first, I did not like the veggie burger yet. Then I liked it a little. And now I like it a lot."

We take this concept a step further by carefully selecting the words we use with children to describe foods. For example, when we first try red and green bell peppers with children, we talk about which is the juiciest and crunchiest and avoid words that imply strong values, such as *the best* and *the worst*. If a child chooses to use one of these words, we respond by saying

"You do not like it yet? You might like it the next time you try it." This response validates the child's opinion but also sends a clear message that it is important to try foods again and again.

## PROVIDING HEALTHY CHOICES

A common family mealtime conflict between adults and children arises when they negotiate about healthy and not-so-healthy food choices—how much of each food can be eaten and which food must be consumed first. It becomes a miserable meal experience for all involved. Much of the pressure is eliminated when children are provided with several healthy food choices and left to decide how much of each food they will eat. By providing only healthy food choices, we help children listen to their own bodies and make choices that support good nutrition and their need to establish autonomy. Equally important, doing so keeps the table conversation pleasant.

In a healthy-foods-only scenario, child care staff and families choose the foods that are bought, prepared, and served. Adults create a pleasing social environment in which the meal is enjoyed. Children are responsible for what and how much they eat.

## TEACHER AND FAMILIES AS ROLE MODELS

Children's dietary habits are established during early years by family preferences, lifestyle, culture, and experience. As more and more children spend a substantial portion of their day in group care settings, early childhood professionals play an increasingly important role in guiding children's food preferences and eating habits. But how many adults intentionally try to increase children's interest in eating healthy foods through creating a purposeful environment? How many adults regularly engage children in the preparation of nutritious foods? How many adults regularly ponder how to incorporate healthy foods and

---

**EARLY SPROUTS TASTING SUGGESTIONS FOR TEACHERS AND FAMILIES**

Always eat a portion of the Early Sprouts recipe yourself. Children will be more willing to try the recipe if you are eating it with them.

Invite the children to serve themselves from a common bowl by taking a scoop from it. When a child has finished eating the first scoop, offer him a second helping.

Be a positive role model—be adventurous about trying new things, and encourage children to do the same. Encourage all children to try at least one bite of the recipe.

If you like the recipe, share your enthusiasm and positive comments. If you do not like the recipe, please be discreet. Do not openly criticize the food.

Compliment the children on the food—many of them participated in making it! Thank them for their hard work making delicious food.

Ask the children to explain how they made the food (for example, ingredients, stirring, measuring). They will be proud of their hard work and their recipe.

Talk about pleasant things and discourage the children from talking about unpleasant topics or openly criticizing the food.

nutritious messages into the learning environments of young children? The box on page 24 provides a list of tips for caregivers and families to assist you in creating a nutritionally purposeful environment for eating with young children.

## INCORPORATE THE EARLY SPROUTS FOOD PHILOSOPHY

Allow children to serve themselves an amount they think they can eat. Do not force them to finish everything; rather, remind them to take a smaller portion next time. Talk with children about how people develop a liking for new foods over time. Foods that are provided for lunch and/or snack should be nutritionally balanced. Follow the principles of reduced fat, sugar, and salt in all the foods you serve. Work to increase fruit, vegetable, and whole grain consumption. On days when an Early Sprouts food is not served as snack, provide vegetables or fruit along with a whole grain cereal or cracker for snack. For birthday celebrations, ask children to chose between scone and muffin recipes for their birthday treat. (You can cook either in a cake pan.) Children don't need frosting to make a cake feel special. Holiday parties (if celebrated in your center) can also incorporate Early Sprouts recipes. Vegetables or fruit with dip, Zucchini Oatmeal Cookies, or Vegetable Quesadillas are some examples of healthy finger foods for classroom parties.

Work to support your entire staff and children's families in accepting and modeling the same food philosophy. Teachers and other staff members should demonstrate an adventurous spirit and be willing to taste new foods. Invite adults to sit down and join the children for snacks and meals. Enthusiastic adults encourage children to try cooking activities and other food explorations. Children are quick to notice the teacher who consumes a soda during naptime, the one who runs in and out of the classroom to consume her morning coffee and donut, and the one who never eats the Early Sprouts foods. They are equally quick to respond to the teacher who displays enthusiasm for fruits, vegetables, and whole grains, eats bell peppers and carrot sticks at lunch, and eagerly tries each new Early Sprouts recipe. Providing consistency in children's exposures to food can set the stage for a lifetime of healthy eating.

Model the Early Sprouts philosophy for families and communicate your approach to food clearly. This is important in promoting positive eating habits. Through Early Sprouts, we can help families overcome their own fears about new foods. We can remind them of the importance of modeling healthy eating habits for their children. We can teach them that everyone

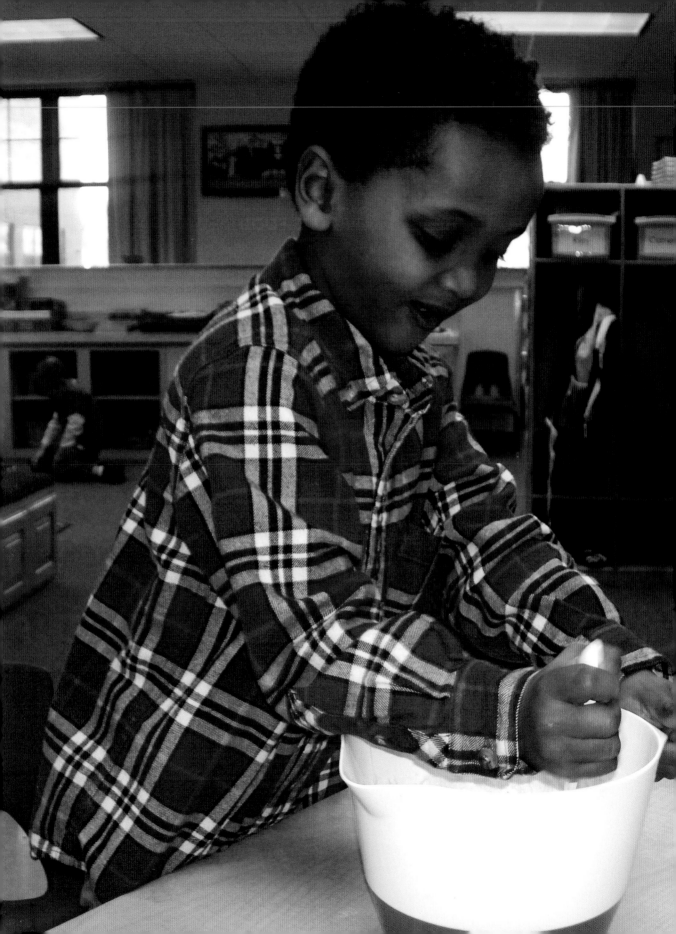

—◆—

# THREE

# EARLY SPROUTS AND THE EARLY LEARNING GUIDELINES

Do you remember the joy of learning something for the first time? Maybe it was riding a two-wheel bike or learning to tie your shoes. Do you remember the cool feeling of snowflakes on your cheeks as they fell from the sky and you tried to catch them on your tongue, or the warmth of the sun on your skin on a hot summer day before you jumped into the pool? How about the taste of a freshly picked apple as you walked through an orchard in autumn? Young children experience those feelings every day. There is an excitement and joy in everything the world has to offer. When we as adults engage in the world of young children, we can enjoy their spirit of adventure and share in their joyful journey of learning.

On this journey, the National Association for the Education of Young Children (NAEYC) provides early childhood educators with resources for creating learning environments based on child development. Educators support children through relationships with responsive adults; active, hands-on involvement; and meaningful experiences and opportunities to construct their understanding of the world (Copple and Bredekamp 2009). The National Association was founded in 1926 and is currently the world's largest nonprofit organization working on the behalf of children. According to its website, NAEYC "is dedicated to improving the well-being of all young children with particular focus on the quality of educational and developmental services for all children birth through age eight."

The Association's *Developmentally Appropriate Practice in Early Childhood Programs Serving Children from Birth through Age 8: A Position Statement of the National Association for the Education of Young Children* (NAEYC 2009, 1) defines developmentally appropriate practice in its 2009 position statement, which reads in part:

The purpose of this position statement is to promote excellence in early childhood education by providing a framework for best practice. Grounded both in the research on child development and learning and in the knowledge base regarding educational effectiveness, the framework outlines practices that promote young children's optimal learning and development. Since its first adoption in 1986, this framework has been known as developmentally appropriate practice. . . .

This statement is intended to complement NAEYC's other position statements on practice, which include *Early Learning Standards* and *Early Childhood Curriculum, Assessment, and Program Evaluation*, as well as the *Code of Ethical Conduct and NAEYC Early Childhood Program Standards and Accreditation Criteria*.

For more information on developmentally appropriate practice, visit www.naeyc.org/dap.

Head Start is a program of the United States Department of Health and Human Services that provides comprehensive education, health, nutrition, and parent involvement services to low-income children and their families. The Head Start program began in 1965 and was later updated by the Head Start Act of 1981. Its most intense revisions occurred in the December 2007 reauthorization. Teachers planning curriculum in Head Start Programs use the Head Start Child Development and Early Learning Framework as one of their guidelines. This framework includes the following domains:

- physical development and health

- social and emotional development

- approaches to learning

- logic and reasoning

- language development

- English language development

- literacy knowledge and skills

- mathematics knowledge and skills

- science knowledge and skills

- creative arts expression

- social studies knowledge and skills

## Fig. 2    THE HEAD START CHILD DEVELOPMENT AND EARLY LEARNING FRAMEWORK

These domains △ and domain elements ▶ apply to all 3 to 5 year olds in Head Start and other early childhood programs, including dual language learners and children with disabilities.

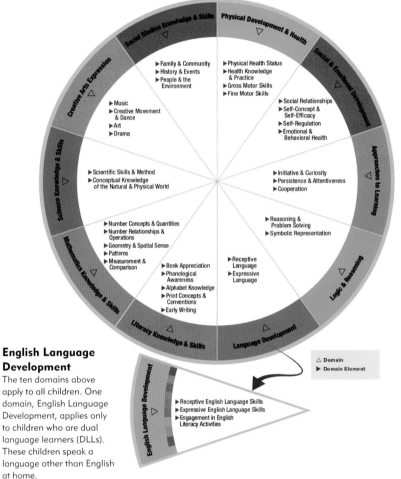

**English Language Development**

The ten domains above apply to all children. One domain, English Language Development, applies only to children who are dual language learners (DLLs). These children speak a language other than English at home.

Most recently, all of the fifty states and the District of Columbia have developed State Early Learning Guidelines (ELGs). These contain statements that specify developmental expectations for preschool children and address traditional content areas, including math, science, and literacy. They also include social-emotional and physical development as well as approaches to learning. The *process* of learning is a critical component of early childhood education. Education for young children is about acquiring and refining foundational skills that will support content learning as children grow. As

ELGs are incorporated into early childhood teaching practice, you want to retain the philosophy and practices outlined by NAEYC. Developmentally appropriate practice (DAP) is based on the knowledge of how young children develop and learn. Early childhood educators engage in a process of making decisions about the well-being and education of the young children in their care, including these five key aspects of good teaching:

1. Creating a caring community of learners

2. Teaching to enhance development and learning

3. Planning appropriate curriculum

4. Assessing children's development and learning

5. Developing reciprocal relationships with families

ELGs that are broad and flexible provide opportunities for authentic assessment of children's growth and development. Good early childhood practices incorporate learning, academics, and standards into play with purpose and intent. Observing and interacting with children in play and relating those experiences to standards is in line with NAEYC's position on assessment. Assessment practices include teacher observation notes, children's work samples, and photographs. Using the ELGs to evaluate the child's growth and development, based on observations and work samples, can provide thoughtful early educators with a comprehensive understanding of individual children. They can also provide opportunities for curriculum assessment and help early educators to make children's learning more visible.

Visible learning is evident in Early Sprouts cooking activities when children wash their hands before cooking (health and safety), take turns (social-emotional development), crack open eggs (approaches to learning), use wooden spoons to mix ingredients (physical development), and count the number of ingredients in a recipe (cognitive). Keeping the ELGs in mind as you work with children in Early Sprouts and other activities shows you how children are moving toward those goals and growing through those hands-on activities. To find the early learning guidelines for your state, you can go to the National Child Care Information and Technical Assistance Center, Department of Health and Human Services Administration for Children and Families, http://nccic.acf.hhs.gov/resource/state-early-learning guidelines.

Teachers who value an emergent curriculum (Jones and Nimmo 1994) or the project approach to learning (Cadwell 1997; Katz and Chard 2000) have found that incorporating the Early Sprouts approach into their classroom stimulates children's thinking. It also provides many new ideas for projects.

Children's questions about plant growth, taste sensations, and cooking processes lead to deeper knowledge of science, math, and the natural world. Children's creative explorations lead to artwork, dramatization, stories, and songs that express their ideas about healthy foods. Cassie, a pre-K teacher whose classroom has implemented the program, says, "From the perspective of an early childhood teacher, this program is very holistic. It's not isolated to an Early Sprouts table. It allows us to do everything."

The Early Sprouts approach, including its focus on cooking with young children, supports the growth and development of young children in developmentally appropriate ways, and it is compatible with Head Start Program Standards and State Early Learning Guidelines. Early childhood education is focused on supporting children's growth and development in the areas of social-emotional, cognitive, health and physical, language and communication, and creative arts development, as well as approaches to learning.

Children learn through experience and hands-on activity. Early childhood educators create an environment for children to explore and build their knowledge. Teachers observe and guide children, and early childhood teachers know that an integrated approach to learning is most effective with young children. We can see the impact it has on teachers and families when we explore issues of nutrition and health.

Early Sprouts is grounded in sound nutritional principles as well as in child development theory. Its goal is to increase consumption of healthy foods through a positive, engaging, and developmentally appropriate curriculum. Early Sprouts recognizes the importance of the roles of families and teachers in the lives of children. It supports adults as they learn with children to enjoy healthy eating habits.

## APPROACHES TO LEARNING

Early childhood theory recognizes the important role of play in young children's development. In developing ELGs, many states have included learning domain as a category along with physical, cognitive, social-emotional, creative expression/aesthetic, communication and literacy development and health/safety. In the New Hampshire Early Learning Guidelines, the focus of the approach to learning domain is on the child's development and use of problem-solving strategies. Five interconnected strands are identified within this domain, including play, learning styles, risk taking, engagement, and reflection. The Early Sprouts approach embraces children's enthusiasm for learning and supports their engagement in it. Our approach also recognizes the importance of adults in guiding children's learning.

Environmentalist Rachel Carson was fascinated by how young children discover learning and the responsibility of adults in their lives. She describes it this way, "If a child is to keep alive his inborn sense of wonder . . . he needs the companionship of at least one adult who can share it, rediscovering with him the joy, excitement and mystery of the world we live in" (Carson 1998, 55).

Children enter the world with a sense of wonder. As early educators, we nurture this enthusiasm for learning and support children's engagement with the world. The Early Sprouts approach encourages children to explore the natural environment, including the foods they eat. Sensory explorations allow teachers to slow down and look at the world through the eyes of the child. In this approach, everyone is present in the process of cooking. Children should have time to ask questions, make comparisons, and share stories. We want to cook the recipe, but we also want to support children's curiosity and sense of wonder.

. . . . . . . . . . . . . . . . . . . . . . . . . . . . . .
## COGNITIVE DEVELOPMENT

Cognitive development refers to the mind and how it works. It involves how children think, how they see their world, and how they use what they learn (Dodge, Colker, and Heroman 2002, 21). The world is an exciting place for children. As we interact with them, we support their enthusiasm and their engagement in learning. Hands-on experiences with fruits and vegetables and cooking activities invites young children to use the traditional five senses—sight, hearing, touch, smell, and taste—as well as their perceptions of temperature, body awareness, and kinesthetic sense, known as *proprioception*. Each of these senses contributes the children's knowledge of foods. The Early Sprouts approach provides multiple opportunities for children to develop cognitive skills by participating in focused scientific exploration.

With repeated exposure to foods, children can build on their knowledge. They observe, investigate, ask questions, and make comparisons. Children happily proclaim, "Look—I am a scientist" as they engage in sensory exploration. We encourage them to use scientific tools such as magnifying glasses. As teachers work with young children, their questions and observations extend the children's enthusiasm and engagement. Asking questions is an important part of the learning process and encourages children to begin to make predictions. The teacher may ask, "What do you think we will find when we cut open the pepper?" The first time children cut open a bell pepper, they exclaim, as Lizzy did, "Ooh look, there are seeds inside!" The next time, they may have an observation like Nick's when he opened a pepper and noticed the space on the inside: "The pepper is like a house." With repeated exposures, children can move beyond their initial exploration of food and begin to develop particular knowledge of it. Children began to make estimations of the number of seeds inside the peppers. "I think there are 100!" exclaimed Marcus.

Children can extend their cognitive skills by comparing the seeds of a variety of vegetables and fruits. They can count the seeds found in one bean pod and those found in a butternut squash. It is difficult to count the seeds in a tomato or a bell pepper, and by the way—"Where are the seeds inside carrots or Swiss chard?" asked Luke. Investigating seeds can be a provocation that leads to multiple science and math investigations. As you work with children, it is important to listen carefully to their thoughts and ideas. You can take photographs of children engaged in the work and display them to support their explorations. Children can document their own work by drawing what they see and dictating their observations to you.

Cognitive development engages children in the work of science, math, and linguistic development. It is important to provide opportunities for children to construct meaning by problem solving with peers and by developing and testing their assumptions. Cooking presents a wonderful opportunity to learn about cause and effect. Engaging in explorations with all of their senses offers children focused and developmentally appropriate experiences. They can look, touch, smell, listen, and taste as they cook. They can measure and count. They learn that there is a specific sequence to the steps in the recipe that need to be followed. Mathematical concepts are a part of every recipe.

## HEALTH AND NUTRITION CURRICULUM

Health and nutrition is an important domain in early childhood education but one that has often been isolated from other domains. The Early Sprouts approach seeks to integrate health and nutrition into the early childhood curriculum. As children prepare food for their classroom community to share, they are participating in one of the daily needs of the group. Playing this role of caring for the community can be very empowering for them. Eating healthy foods can help them explore the connection between these foods and feeling stronger and better able to concentrate on their work.

When we look at the goals for young children in this area of development, we need to think about the impact of these early years on lifelong habits. These are important years for children to learn good nutrition, hygiene, self-help, and safety practices, all components of a healthy lifestyle.

The Early Sprouts approach includes recipes that are healthy—low in fat, with no added sugars, and that incorporate whole grains. Children are consistently encouraged to explore the ingredients of the recipes, and adults are encouraged to share information on the nutrient value of the foods. In Julie's preschool classroom, she asked the children why they were served vegetables at the snack table. The children replied, "Because we like them, and they are good for you!" The Early Sprouts approach takes a positive attitude toward eating healthy foods. Children investigate the vegetables and construct their own knowledge about them. They ask questions and compare their experiences. As children and teachers cook together, you may ask, "Does the cooked bell pepper taste different than the raw one?" or "What words would you use to describe the difference between the cooked and the raw peppers?" Adults provide children with information about the vegetables while engaged in the cooking activity. As children worked with Swiss chard at one Early Sprouts table, the teacher asked, "Can you think of another vegetable that looks like chard?" Children responded, "Spinach and kale." Then a discussion ensued about green leafy vegetables, the nutrients they offer, and the variety of ways they can be eaten. When early childhood classrooms begin to cook healthy meals and snacks on a consistent basis, amazing opportunities arise for learning healthy eating habits.

The National Association for the Education of Young Children addresses the issue in the following curriculum standard:

> NAEYC Standard 2.K: Curriculum Content Area for Cognitive Development: Health and Safety
>
> 2.K.01 Children are provided varied opportunities and materials that encourage good health practices such as serving and feeding themselves, rest, good nutrition, exercise, hand washing, and tooth brushing.
>
> 2.K.02 Children are provided varied opportunities and materials to help them learn about nutrition, including identifying sources of food and recognizing, preparing, eating, and valuing healthy foods (NAEYC 2006, 26).

## PHYSICAL DEVELOPMENT

Focus on physical development in the preschool years emphasizes body awareness and control and large- and small-muscle development and coordination. Cooking with young children provides multiple opportunities for children to use their eyes and hands together to accomplish fine-motor tasks. Manipulating measuring cups and spoons initially can be a challenge for children. They are excited to learn how to use a straight edge to level off flour in dry measuring cups. We use serrated table knives to cut vegetables. Using a knife safely is a skill that takes practice for most young children, and they are proud when they can accomplish it. Families are often surprised that children use knives in an Early Sprout classroom. (Chapter 4 addresses safety when cooking with young children.)

We believe children are competent and capable beings and that with proper instruction and adult guidance, they can master many kitchen tasks. At ages two to three years, children can learn to stir and mix, shake, spread, scrub, tear, break, or snap vegetables, including lettuce and green beans, and knead bread with adult support. They can also use basic cooking tools, such as whisks, basters, spatulas, strainers, colanders, and cookie cutters. At age three, children become more capable of pouring fluids. It is appropriate to encourage them to use small pitchers at snack and lunch to pour their own milk or water. In cooking activities, they are ready to start pouring liquid ingredients with adult supervision. As the three-year-olds grow toward four, they become ready for more experience with cutting soft foods with knives and using nonelectric appliances, such as juicers or eggbeaters. At four, children are excited to master cracking eggs, cutting harder foods with knives, and mashing. As they become more experienced and capable, they may use graters and vegetable peelers (Colker 2005). These tools can have sharp edges, and adult supervision is important for everyone's safety. Kitchen scissors are a necessary piece of kitchen equipment, and cutting green leafy vegetables with scissors is very rewarding for children. Children in the group who rarely join art activities that use scissors may find that helping to prepare food is a developmentally appropriate way to practice this skill.

## COMMUNICATION AND LANGUAGE

During the preschool years, children are developing their skills in language and communication. Every day they are building their vocabulary and expressive and receptive language skills and laying the groundwork for reading. Cooking activities provide multiple opportunities for communication and language development.

- Expressive language: "The tomato splashed in my face. It is really juicy!"

- Building vocabulary: Cooking has its own terminology, and children are excited to learn new words. Vocabulary development involves a wide range of cooking terms, including *bake, boil, knead, chop,* as well as cooking equipment—*whisk, grater, colander.*

- Retelling the process: This is what Nora had to say when asked about making the muffins for snack: "First we read the recipe. Molly started with measuring the cornmeal. Margo added the yogurt. Then we all helped with the other ingredients. While Sophia stirred the batter, Matthew added the peppers. Margo and I worked as a team to fill the muffin pans. We baked them in the oven and yummy—they are delicious."

- Emergent and early reading: The use of illustrated recipes builds children's awareness of print and the role it plays in society. Children begin to look confidently at the recipe and say, "See, it says 2 cups of flour."

- Listening comprehension: As children work with adults to cook a recipe, they are listening to directions and following a sequence of steps. Annabelle looks to Brian as he joins the cooking table: "The teacher said first we have to chop the tomatoes." She understands that this is the first step in making the Zucchini and Tomato Egg Casserole.

Extension activities can include reading picture books featuring cooking- and nutrition-related concepts. Children can write their own stories. In one early childhood classroom, children took on the challenge of creating a book based on Eric Carle's *Today Is Monday*. In the book, each day of the week has a certain food associated with it. Monday is string beans, Tuesday is spaghetti, Wednesday is soup, and so on. These children created an Early Sprouts version of the book with illustrations based on the original six Early Sprouts vegetables for six days of the week. On Sunday they decided to have smoothies. Before starting the Early Sprouts program, the children had not been served smoothies before. As they began making smoothies regularly, the food quickly became a favorite snack.

## SOCIAL AND EMOTIONAL DEVELOPMENT

The social-emotional domain includes children's understanding of their own emotions and learning to regulate them appropriately. It also involves their developing sense of self and how that self interacts with others. Socially, preschoolers are interested in connecting with their peers and adults. Being part of the classroom community is important to them. They are developing their skills and need the guidance of thoughtful adults to navigate this area of development. Cooking activities provide rich opportunities for them to work together to prepare delicious food that will be enjoyed by their classroom community.

As you cook with children, they engage in conversations that include ingredients, equipment, and tools, as well as thoughts and feelings about what is being accomplished. Children will often share other information about family events and experiences or just something that is on their mind. In *The Cooking Book*, Laura J. Colker writes this:

> Research underscores the importance of adult-child conversations during mealtimes in building vocabulary and literacy skills. Parents can use cooking times as opportunities to talk with children about their own experiences with cooking and to predict what will happen as they cook. Moreover, chatting together while cooking is also an excellent way to strengthen the parent-child bond. And as they cook with their parents, children become more competent and proud to be contributing members of their family (Colker 2005, 50).

Cooking is an activity in which children participate the same way adults do. It is very empowering for them to engage in the real work of preparing a snack or a meal. They take on this challenge with enthusiasm, and with the guidance of a thoughtful adult, they become more competent and capable in the kitchen and beyond. One family member commented, "She loves to cook. So now she wants to cook breakfast with me, lunch with me—I mean, she wants to be in the kitchen whenever we are cooking! She wants to help with everything." Developing this sense of competence is an important social-emotional goal for the preschool child.

As children work with kitchen tools, they become more confident about their abilities. They often help each other. Molly was trying to cut open a cherry tomato with a knife. Bobby was sitting next to her and noticed her struggle. He leaned over and asked, "Do you want me to show you how I did it?" Molly looked up at him and said, "Yes." Bobby proceeded to explain how he held the tomato and how he used his knife. Molly followed his instructions and proudly exclaimed, "I did it!" In the Early Sprout approach, adults are consistently cooking in the classroom with children. They work cooperatively with their peers and the adults in the classroom. This helps them develop their skills in social interactions as well as in other areas of development. Some children are very hesitant about cracking open an egg. Some children may choose to watch other children and adults crack eggs and learn through observation. It is also helpful to have an extra egg or two on hand just in case. Occasionally an egg might hit the floor instead of the mixing bowl. It is important to let children know that mistakes happen and that the situation can be easily resolved. Cracking eggs takes practice, and with the guidance of a supportive adult and peers, children can grow in their competence and joyfully celebrate the day that they can crack an egg with confidence.

The work of cooking supports children's social-emotional development by providing experiences that increase their comfort with new experiences. Cooking consistently gives them the opportunity to reflect on their experiences and apply knowledge to new activities. Often when you are cooking with children, you will hear exclamations of "I did it!" This may come after successfully cracking an egg or carefully measuring the flour and adding it to the mixing bowl. Children are proud of their accomplishments and eager to take on new challenges after they experience these successes. Through their interactions with peers and adults, children build their knowledge of self and others. They begin to articulate their thoughts and ideas and share stories.

The Early Sprouts approach also looks at the importance of family-style meals and snacks. When you eat with children, you model positive and respectful attitudes about foods. The Early Sprouts approach uses the language "I don't like it yet" purposefully. Children are encouraged to share their cooking activities and stories from home about cooking and food. We are always respectful of foods from a variety of cultures and of everyone's preferences and food choices. (In chapter 2, you will find a sidebar entitled "Early Sprouts Tasting Suggestions for Teacher and Families.")

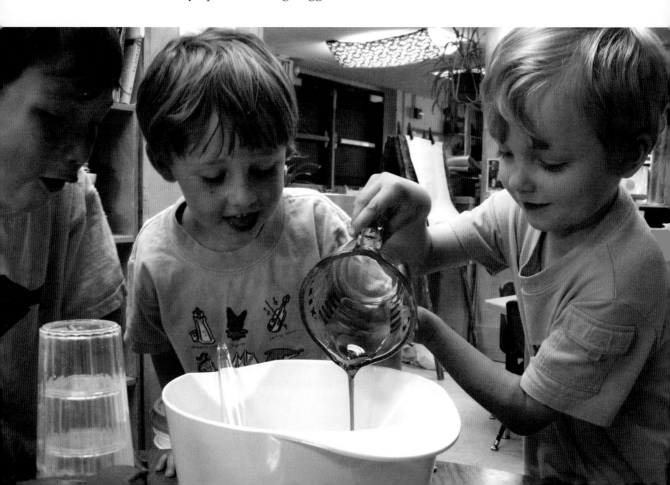

## CONCLUSION

Creating a nutritionally purposeful environment is part of a comprehensive approach to fighting the obesity epidemic. It provides a healthy atmosphere in which children can learn and grow. At home this may be reflected by the presence of healthy snack foods, such as fresh fruit, and the absence of foods high in sugar or salt, such as cookies and potato chips. Adults are strong role models in this approach. You must model healthy practices to children by your behavior and intentional use of language. You should participate with children in healthy eating. Meals at home as well as in the classroom should reflect healthy practices for everyone participating. The Early Sprouts approach provides children with multiple exposures to healthy foods (especially vegetables) with the goal of increasing consumption of them. Sensory exploration activities and cooking experiences for young children help in this. It is important for you and the children's parents to be purposeful in creating environments that reflect healthy practices.

- Dramatic play area foods reflect healthy practices by including fruits and vegetables and multiethnic selections, including sushi rolls, steamed dumplings, and tortillas. Avoid cakes and ice cream.

- Creative dramatic play props are focused on the farmers' market and the doctor's office instead of the ice cream store and candy shop.

- Math manipulatives include counters, such as fruits and vegetables instead of cookies and candies (check out catalogs for ideas).

- Sing songs about healthy practices instead of songs about bubblegum and sugary treats.

- Focus literacy activities on books that convey positive nutrition messages. (See the booklist included in the appendix.)

Take some time to evaluate the cooking area in your early childhood setting for its support of healthy practices and nutritional purposefulness. Review DAP and the ELGs for your state as you plan your curriculum. If you are affiliated with a Head Start program, review the curriculum's goals and standards. The Early Sprouts approach can easily become part of your program and community. It will help you to support the healthy growth and development of the children in your care.

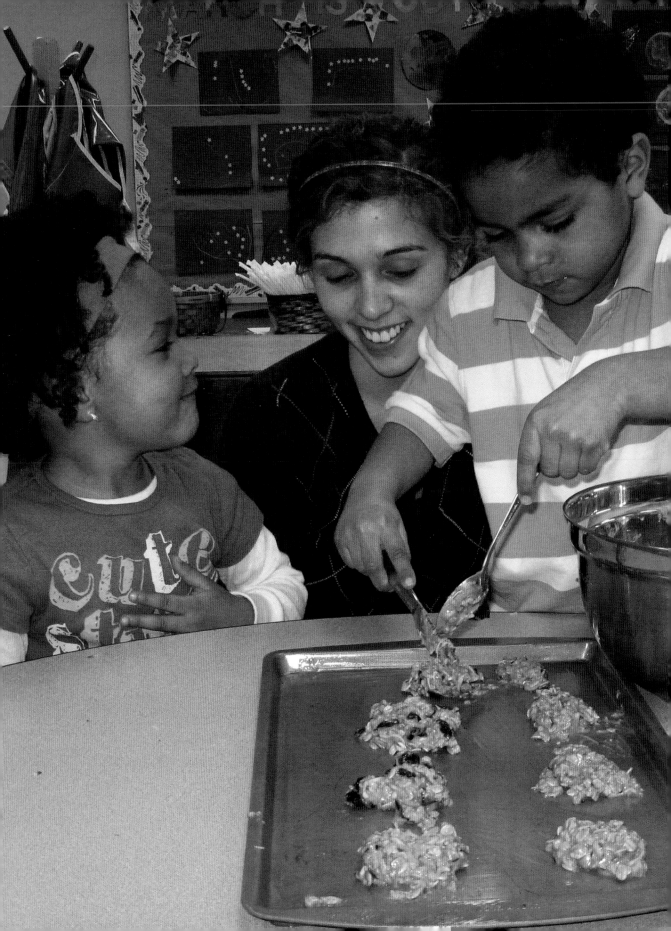

—ᴡᴡ—

# COOKING
# WITH
# YOUNG CHILDREN

Cooking with preschool children can be one of the most rewarding aspects of the classroom curriculum. Young children are naturally curious about the world around them. Cooking activities provide them with the opportunity to engage directly in the real work of preparing food. They are excited to practice new skills and work with grown-up tools, including measuring cups and wire whisks. The cooperative social atmosphere of working together to make food for the classroom community is very engaging to children. While this is an exciting and educational classroom experience for them, it does take some extra preparation and safety precautions on your part.

## CREATE A CHILD-FRIENDLY COOKING ENVIRONMENT

When cooking with children, you need to assess the suitability of your space for the size and skills of the children. Kitchen spaces are built with counters at adult height and storage areas that are out of children's reach. Think about how you can organize the kitchen so children can independently reach simple tools, including measuring cups and spoons, mixing bowls, and wooden spoons.

If you are creating a cooking space in a classroom, try to position it near a sink so children can wash their hands and draw water for cooking. It is helpful if the cooking space is out of the main traffic pattern of the classroom so that cooking activities are not interrupted by other activities. Access to electrical outlets is also important for small appliances, such as an electric frying pan or a portable burner.

Storage of materials is another issue to consider. It is helpful to have low, open shelves so children can see the materials and participate in collecting items for cooking. You may want to label the shelves so children can begin to associate the written name with the equipment. It is also great to have a small refrigerator and perhaps a small convection/microwave oven available in your cooking area. The workspace should be set up with emphases on safety, how children move through the space, and how adults interact with children in the space. Beautiful space is more engaging to work in, so think about how to organize the area so it appeals to you and the children. If you are cooking with children in a family child care setting, keep safety in mind and consider how you can reorganize your kitchen to make it more user-friendly for children.

## COLLECTING THE TOOLS

Cooking in the classroom requires the same basic equipment you use at home to prepare recipes. Here are the cooking items we recommend for Early Sprouts cooking:

### General Kitchen Items

| | |
|---|---|
| baking pans | measuring cups–liquid and dry |
| can opener | measuring spoons |
| colander | mixing bowls |
| cookie sheets | muffin pans |
| cutting boards | peeler |
| grater | potato masher |
| hot pads and oven mitts | spatula |
| kitchen parchment | vegetable brushes |
| kitchen scissors | wooden mixing spoons |
| knives | whisk |

### Small Appliances

| | |
|---|---|
| blender | portable electric griddle |
| food processor | portable electric skillet |
| mini convection oven | toaster |
| portable burner | |

## SAFETY CONCERNS

While cooking with children can be a joyful and adventurous experience, it also needs to be safe. Plan the physical environment as well as teach children safe practices. Exercise appropriate supervision at all times, and keep a first-aid kit close by. If a skin burn occurs, remember to treat it by placing the burned area under cold, running water. To keep your cooking area safe follow these precautions:

- Make sure that sharp knives are stored out of reach of children.

- Check that the electrical outlets are not overloaded.

- Cover unused electrical outlets with safety caps.

- Store cleaning agents out of children's reach.

- Keep your cooking space clean and uncluttered.

- Check that hot pads are dry and without holes.

- Always use hot pads when removing baking dishes from the oven and on handles when removing a pot from the stove.

- Keep pot handles turned to the inside of the stove when you are not stirring.

- When removing a lid from a hot pot, always open and move the lid away from your body and face.

- Use only wooden spoons when stirring in hot pots and pans.

- Make sure your hands are dry before plugging in an appliance.

When you begin cooking with children, set the tone for the activity. Talk with them about how to cook cooperatively. In many Early Sprouts classrooms, the teacher begins turn-taking with one child and then proceeds around the table. With this approach, children know whose turn it is and can anticipate when their own turn is coming. Sometimes you may want to divide one cup of flour into two half cups so more children can have the opportunity to participate. Let them know that cooking is fun but also serious work. Explain that it is important for them to sit safely in their own space. Encourage them to use an appropriate tone and voice level while working. Warn them before you turn on loud appliances, including the blender or food processor. If children know what to expect, they can participate in the work thoughtfully.

Introducing children to equipment and supplies is an important part of the cooking experience. You can teach them the correct name for materials and what each piece of equipment does. Knives, for example, are very important tools for preparing food. Serrated table knives work well for our Early Sprouts recipes. To help children use knives safely, follow these precautions:

- Always hold a knife by the handle, never by the blade.

- Use the serrated edge of a table knife to cut the food.

- When using knives, children should keep their bodies calm and safe.

- Teachers should always be present and attentive when children are cutting.

- Teach children to make the fingers of their noncutting hands into a claw to steady foods for cutting. This keeps their fingers out of the way of the knife blade.

Graters and vegetable peelers have sharp edges. Supervise children's use of these items closely. Make sure to demonstrate to each child how to hold on to foods safely when grating or peeling. Young children are building their fine-muscle coordination and are eager to practice these skills. At ages two to three years, children are developmentally capable of stirring and mixing, shaking, spreading, scrubbing, tearing, breaking or snapping, kneading, and using basic cooking gadgets, including whisks, spatulas, strainers, and colanders. At ages three to four years, children are ready to pour, roll (with a rolling pin or their hands), measure ingredients into cups and spoons, cut soft foods, and use nonelectric appliances (for example, a beater or a juicer) with adult supervision. At age four years, children are excited to crack eggs, assist with using electrical appliances (blender, mixer, electric frying pan), use a knife with adult supervision, and mash. At ages four to five years, they can grate with adult supervision.

## CLEANUP AND SETUP

Cooking with young children can become messy. They are just beginning to build the fine-motor coordination that allows them to measure a cup of flour. Pouring and dumping are not yet refined skills. Encourage them to do their best. They should take cooking projects seriously but also recognize that spills sometimes happen. Always include children in cleaning up any spills, and reassure them that grown-ups have accidents too. Be relaxed and supportive as you teach children how to wipe up a spill at the table or sweep up flour from the floor. Encourage children to help each other by clearly defining their tasks. "Jacob, you can sweep the floor with the broom, and Elizabeth can hold the dustpan." Building cooperative work skills is an important focus for all preschool children. Young children already love water play. Take advantage of this interest to encourage them to help with cooking cleanup. It is easy to fill a sink with warm, soapy water, pull a stool up to the sink, and let children get to work. Remember that your attitude is important: if you present cleanup tasks as dreary and dreadful, children may take on that attitude too. Be positive and encouraging about cleanup and see how children respond. Here's a list of some cleaning materials you may want to have available for children:

- small brooms and dustpans
- dishpan and drainer

- mop

- paper towels

- sponges

After your area and the equipment you need are set up, prepare for the specific recipe. Cooking with children requires the extra step of planning their experience. As you read through the recipe, think about how the children can be involved. Can they help wash the vegetables for the recipe? How many children can you comfortably supervise with knives while they cut apples? If the dish needs to bake for 1 hour and 10 minutes and then cool before eating, how does that lengthy cooking time affect the rest of your schedule?

- Read through the recipe.

- Check the ingredients list and collect everything.

- Make sure you have the necessary equipment available.

- Check the time needed for this recipe.

- Plan children's engagement in the work. What will they do?

- Plan a serving time for the food.

Once you feel your space is prepared and you have chosen a recipe, it is time to engage children in the work. Make sure the table is clean and sanitized and that everyone has washed hands before cooking. Remember—your attitude is important. Present the recipe to children enthusiastically. Be creative in your invitation. For example, you might read *Red Are the Apples* with the children before making the Apple Snack Cake. Hide the cauliflower in a feely bag and ask children to identify it by feel. Give them opportunities to guess before beginning to make the Roasted Cauliflower. It is possible that you do not like cauliflower yet. We have found that many adults have not tasted roasted cauliflower and are surprised at how much they like it once they taste it. It is important that you taste the Early Sprouts recipe along with the children. Refer to the tasting suggestions in chapter 2. Remember to use language intentionally. It is okay for you to say, "I don't like it yet." Teachers need to keep tasting the recipes along with the children. It is amazing how the world of healthy eating really will open up for you!

Cooking with young children is a rich experience. It takes thoughtful planning and careful supervision, but the benefits are worth it. Cooking offers children the opportunity to practice skills and begin to learn lifelong, healthy eating habits.

# FIVE

# BREAKFAST
# RECIPES

W E ARE CERTAINLY NOT THE FIRST to tell you that breakfast is the most important meal of the day (though the others are important too!). Breakfast breaks the overnight fast—hence the word *break-fast*—and revs up our metabolism. Children and adults who eat a nutritious, well-balanced breakfast focus and learn better than those who are non–breakfast eaters. Children who consume a healthy breakfast also tend to exhibit better behavior. Breakfast eaters are more successful in maintaining healthy body weight. Finally, breakfast eaters report being happier and experiencing overall feelings of well-being.

Choosing a healthy breakfast does not always come easily to Americans. Our traditional morning meals often consist of bacon, greasy eggs, hash browns, and buttered white toast. In this chapter, we provide recipes that offer a healthier, more-balanced approach to start the children's day. The recipes are rich in whole grains, dietary fiber, fruits, vegetables, healthy oils, and flavor. The Child and Adult Care Food Program (CACFP) requires three breakfast components for children ages three to five years:

1. ¾ cup of fluid milk

2. ½ cup of vegetables, fruit, or 100 percent juice

3. ½ slice bread (enriched or whole grain),
   ⅓ cup cold cereal (enriched or whole grain),
   ¼ cup hot cereal (enriched or whole grain), or
   ¼ cup cooked pasta or noodle products

Our recipes fulfill one to two of these CACFP breakfast components with a note in the nutrition information section that guides you in easily meeting the remaining requirements.

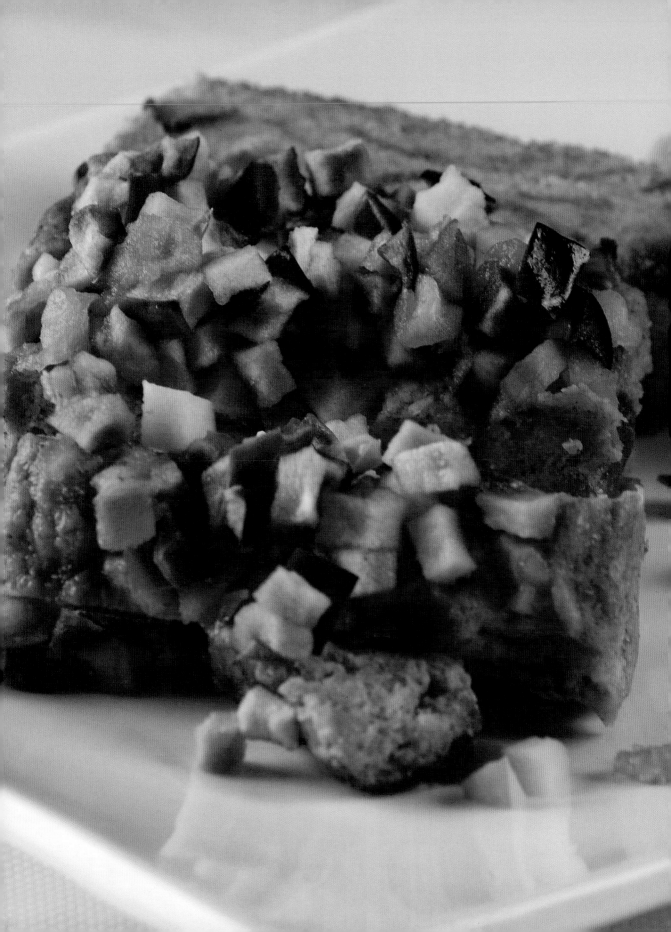

# *Baked Apple French Toast Squares*

Estimated preparation and cooking time: 50 minutes

## INGREDIENTS

5 large eggs

¾ cup skim milk

1½ teaspoons ground cinnamon, divided into ½ teaspoon and 1 teaspoon

1 teaspoon vanilla extract

10 slices whole wheat bread

5 tablespoons pure maple syrup

5 apples, medium to large

## PROCEDURE

1. **Preheat oven to 350°F and line a 9 x 13-inch baking pan with parchment.**
2. **In large bowl, whisk together eggs, milk, ½ teaspoon cinnamon, and vanilla.**
3. **Cut or tear bread into small cubes and add to egg mixture. Mix gently until all bread pieces are coated. Spread mixture evenly in baking pan and set aside.**
4. **Peel and cut apples into bite-sized pieces. Pour maple syrup into large microwavable bowl and microwave 20 seconds. Add 1 teaspoon cinnamon and mix well. Add apples to syrup and toss until all pieces are coated. Spread apple mixture evenly over bread.**
5. **Bake 35 minutes or until apples are softened and bread pieces are firm. Cool slightly and serve.**

Yield: 10 servings

- **Try making the French Toast Squares with different types of fruit, such as peaches, blueberries, plums, pears, or cherries.**
- **November 28 is National French Toast Day in the United States.**
- **The French have long made a dish of bread that is soaked in eggs and cooked on a griddle, and many other European countries have too. No one knows who first invented it.**
- **In France, the dish is known as *pain perdu*, which translates into English as "lost bread." In England, it used to be called "poor knights pudding," but today it is known as "eggy bread."**

## NUTRITION INFORMATION

Serving size: 1/10 recipe

Per serving: 180 calories, 3 g total fat, ½ g saturated fat, 90 mg cholesterol, 31 g carbohydrates, 5 g fiber, 17 g sugars, 8 g protein, and 180 mg sodium

CACFP: Serve with ¾ cup fluid milk.

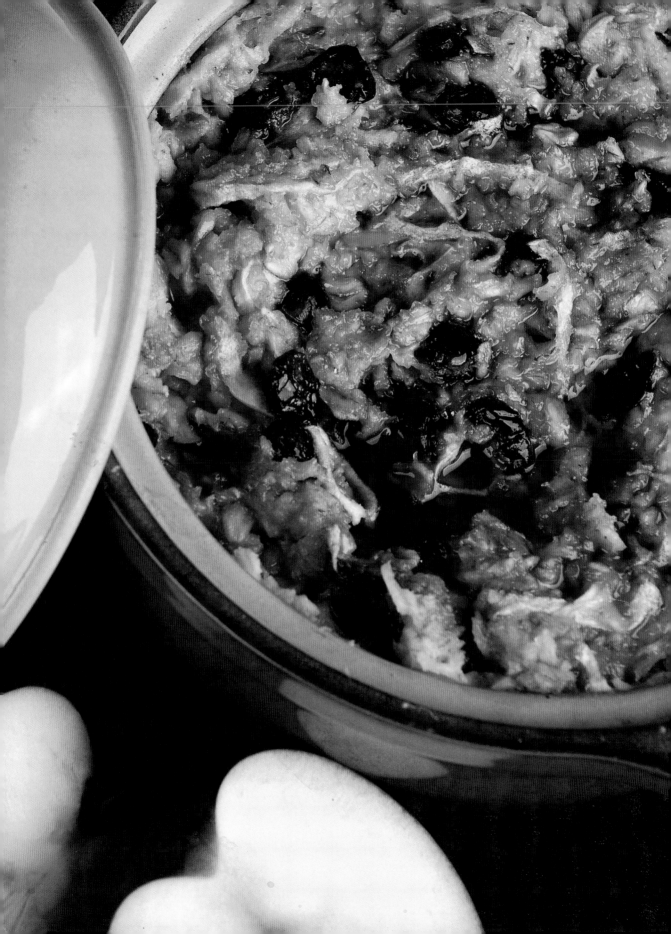

# Apple Baked Oatmeal

Estimated preparation and cooking time: 50 minutes

## INGREDIENTS

3½ cups skim milk

2 cups old-fashioned rolled oats

⅔ cup dried fruit (we used cranberries and snipped apricots)

⅛ teaspoon salt

1 tablespoon pure maple syrup

1 medium apple, peeled and cored

- Other dried fruits, such as raisins, blueberries, and cherries, may be substituted for cranberries and apricots.

- Rolled oats are whole grains that have been steamed and flattened (literally rolled over) so they cook more quickly.

- Oats are a heart-healthy food rich in soluble fiber and antioxidants.

- Be sure to use pure maple syrup. The pancake syrup found in grocery stores is corn syrup based, artificially flavored, and contains little to no real maple syrup.

- Native Americans began making maple syrup well before Europeans came to the New World.

- Up until 1885, maple sugar was less expensive than cane sugar in the United States.

- Baked oatmeal is a popular dish among the Amish. Our version is a slightly healthier twist on this old favorite.

## PROCEDURE

1. Preheat oven to 350°F.

2. In 4-quart microwavable, ovenproof casserole dish, heat milk 1–2 minutes in microwave. Mix in oats and set aside.

3. Snip apricots. Mix apricots, cranberries, salt, and maple syrup into oats and milk mixture. Shred apple and add to casserole dish. Stir until evenly mixed.

4. Bake uncovered 20 minutes. Stir and bake 15 minutes or until oats are chewy.

5. Allow to cool slightly and serve.

Yield: 10 servings

## NUTRITION INFORMATION

Serving size: ¹/₁₀ recipe

Per serving: 160 calories, 1 g total fat, 0 g saturated fat, 0 mg cholesterol, 32 g carbohydrates, 2 g fiber, 12 g sugars, 8 g protein, and 80 mg sodium

CACFP: Serve with ¾ cup fluid milk and ½ cup fruit, such as sliced peaches.

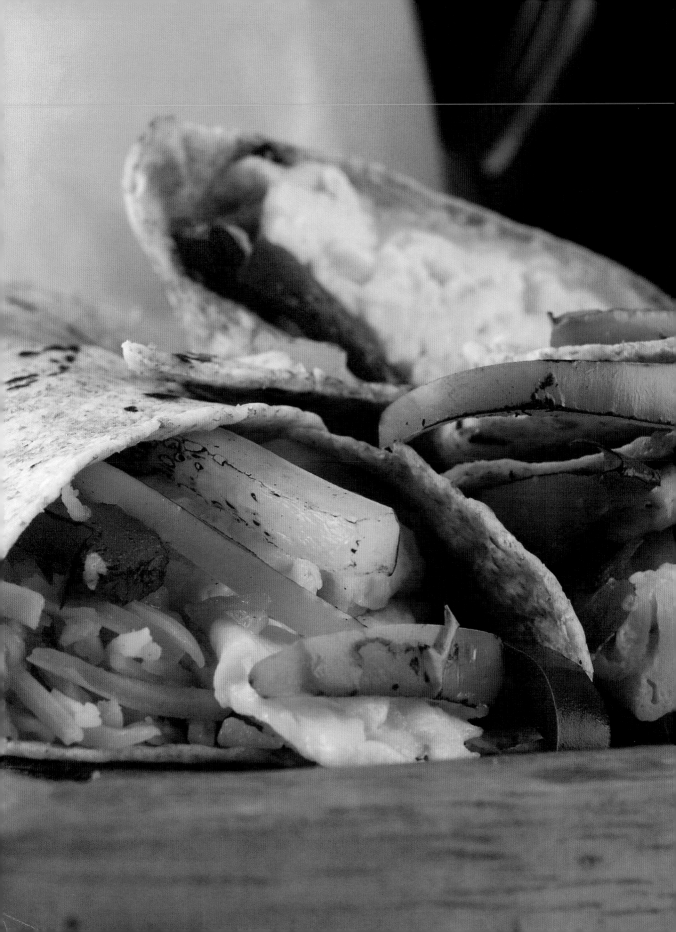

# Bell Pepper Breakfast Burritos

Estimated preparation and cooking time: 25 minutes

## INGREDIENTS

¾ cup shredded sharp cheddar cheese

1½ large red bell peppers

6 large eggs

⅓ cup skim milk

10 whole grain tortillas (6-inch)

Nonstick cooking spray

- ☙ Use red, yellow, and green bell peppers to add extra color and nutrition to your breakfast burritos.

- ☙ Substitute asparagus, spinach, broccoli, cooked sweet potatoes, or black beans for the bell peppers.

- ☙ The carotenoids lutein and zeaxanthin in eggs may help keep our eyes healthy.

- ☙ A single egg contains 6 grams of protein and all of the essential amino acids.

- ☙ No significant link has been established between eggs and heart disease.

- ☙ Eggs are low in cost and easy to prepare.

- ☙ This recipe can also be a great lunch.

- ☙ Tortillas are a good source of whole grains.

## PROCEDURE

1. If not preshredded, grate cheese in food processor or use cheese grater.

2. Seed bell peppers and dice into very small pieces.

3. In large mixing bowl, whisk together eggs and milk.

4. Apply nonstick cooking spray to skillet and preheat to medium-high. Sauté peppers until softened.

5. Add egg mixture to skillet and cook, stirring frequently with rubber spatula. Once eggs start to set, add shredded cheese.

6. Continue to cook (stirring occasionally) until eggs are completely set.

7. Portion egg mixture onto tortillas, roll, and serve.

Yield: 10 burritos

## NUTRITION INFORMATION

Serving size: 1 burrito

Per serving: 230 calories, 8 g total fat, 2 g saturated fat, 115 mg cholesterol, 25 g carbohydrates, 2 g fiber, 3 g sugars, 10 g protein, and 270 mg sodium

CACFP: Serve with ¾ cup fluid milk and ¼ cup fresh fruit (or 100 percent juice).

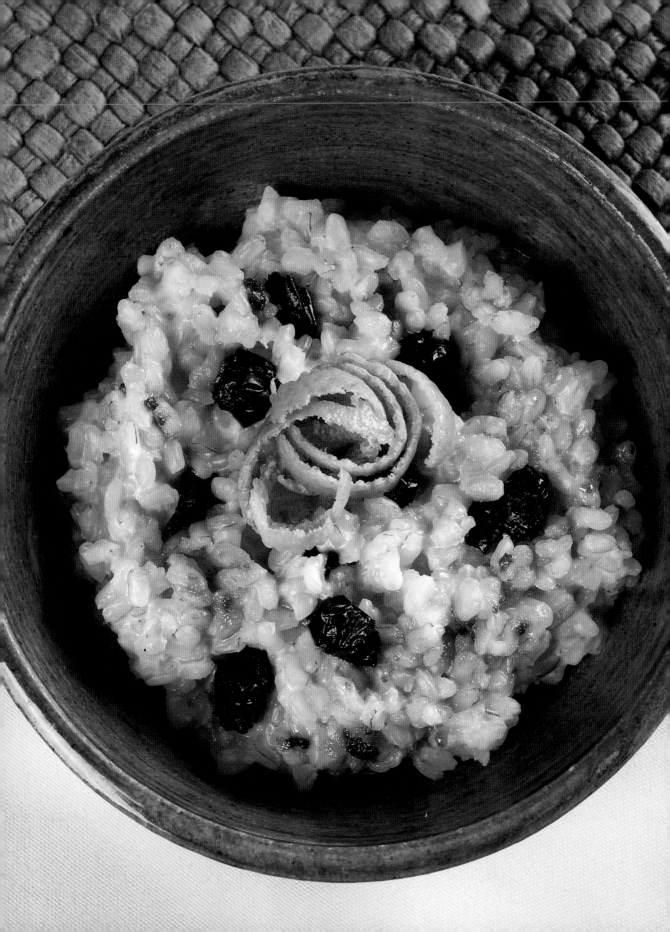

# Creamy Cranberry–Brown Rice Pudding

Estimated preparation and cooking time: 2 days
(1 hour the day before and 20 minutes the day of serving)

## INGREDIENTS

3 wide strips of orange zest

6 cups nonfat milk or water

2 cups raw brown rice

1½ cups skim milk

1 tablespoon brown sugar

1 teaspoon ground cinnamon

½ cup dried cranberries

ϙ People have been eating rice for about 9,000 years. Rice is a staple food for more than 3 billion people—about half of the world's population.

ϙ In some Asian countries, people greet each other, not by saying, "How are you?" but instead by asking "Have you eaten rice today?"

ϙ Brown rice is a whole grain and is more nutritious than white rice. It is rich in vitamins, minerals, fiber, and phytonutrients that are lost when rice is milled and polished.

ϙ The rice plant has many uses. It can be made into beverages, paper, cosmetics, laundry starch, ethanol, construction materials, animal bedding, cooking oil, and glue.

## PROCEDURE

### Day 1

1. Cut three long, wide orange peel strips, using only orange portion of skin.

2. Combine 6 cups milk or water, 3 large orange zest strips, and brown rice in large saucepan, cover, and bring to boil over medium heat.

3. Uncover, reduce heat to medium-low, and simmer 40–50 minutes or until mixture is thickened and rice is tender, stirring frequently to prevent sticking.

4. Remove orange strips and discard.

5. Allow rice to cool; transfer to glass storage container, cover, and store in refrigerator.

### Day 2

1. Transfer rice into large saucepan and add remaining 1½ cups milk, brown sugar, and cinnamon.

2. Cook over medium heat until warm and creamy, about 20 minutes.

3. Add dried cranberries.

4. Allow to cool slightly and serve.

Yield: 10 servings

## NUTRITION INFORMATION

Serving size: ½ cup pudding

Per serving: 230 calories, 0 g total fat, 0 g saturated fat, 5 mg cholesterol, 46 g carbohydrates, 2 g fiber, 14 g sugars, 9 g protein, and 80 mg sodium

CACFP: Serve with ½ cup fresh fruit and ¾ cup fluid milk.

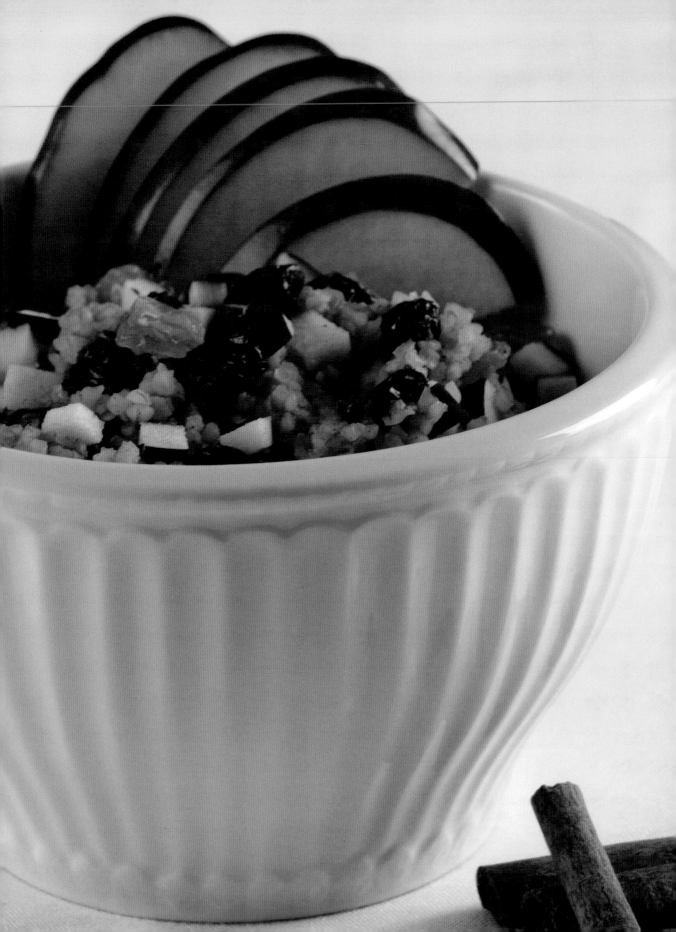

# Hearty Apple & Raisin Cereal

Estimated preparation and cooking time: 30 minutes

## INGREDIENTS

4 apples, medium, diced in
½ inch pieces

1½ cups raisins

2 teaspoons ground cinnamon
(or to taste)

2 cups raw bulgur wheat

4 cups water

2 cups skim milk (heat if desired)

½ cup maple syrup (or to taste)

## PROCEDURE

1.  In small bowl, combine apples, raisins, and cinnamon; set aside.

2.  In medium saucepan, combine bulgur with 4 cups water. Cook on medium-high until soft, about 15 minutes.

3.  Spoon bulgur into large serving bowl. Add milk, maple syrup, and apple mixture. Mix well and serve.

Yield: 10 servings

## NUTRITION INFORMATION

Serving size: ¹/₁₀ recipe

Per serving: 240 calories, ½ g total fat, 0 g saturated fat, 0 mg cholesterol, 59 g carbohydrates, 8 g fiber, 32 g sugars, 6 g protein, and 25 mg sodium

CACFP: Serve with ¾ cup fluid milk.

⸎ Top the cereal with toasted pecans (if your center allows nuts) or granola (see page 61).

⸎ Substitute soy, rice, or almond milk for cow's milk.

⸎ Bulgur contains more fiber, vitamins, and minerals than rice.

⸎ Bulgur is wheat kernels that have been steamed, dried, and crushed. It is made from several different varieties of wheat.

⸎ Bulgur is a staple food in the Middle East and can be found in the natural food section of grocery stores.

⸎ Bulgur can be used in pilafs, breads, and grain-based salads, such as tabbouleh.

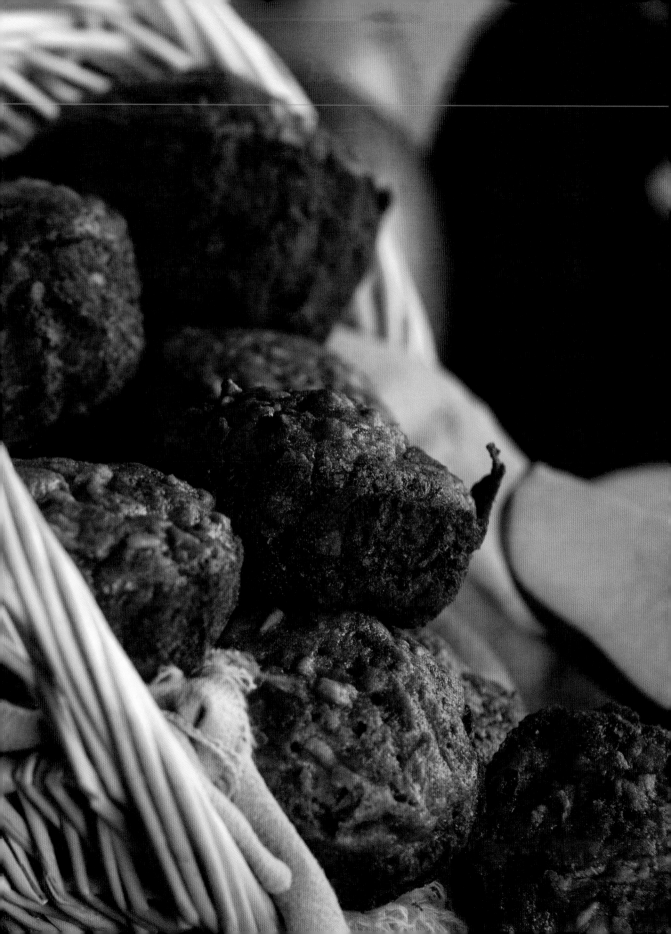

# Harvest Muffins

Estimated preparation and cooking time: 40 minutes

## INGREDIENTS

1 cup white whole wheat flour or whole wheat pastry flour

1 cup rolled oats

½ cup brown sugar

1 tablespoon ground cinnamon

¾ teaspoon baking soda

2 teaspoons baking powder

3 cups finely diced or shredded apples (about 2–3 large apples)

1½ cups shredded carrots

2 eggs

½ cup skim milk

4 tablespoons canola oil

Nonstick cooking spray

⊬ Harvest Muffins are a source of fruit, vegetable, and whole grains.

⊬ Substitute shredded zucchini for the carrots or pears for the apples.

⊬ Add raisins and nuts for a nutritional boost!

⊬ Cinnamon is a perfect spice for the fall and winter. The spice is ground from the bark of the cinnamon tree.

⊬ Ground cinnamon stays fresh for about six months, while cinnamon sticks stay fresh for about a year.

⊬ Cinnamon has been shown to have anticlotting properties and also assists in blood sugar control.

## PROCEDURE

1. Preheat oven to 375°F. Coat muffin pan with nonstick cooking spray.

2. In large bowl, combine flour, oats, brown sugar, cinnamon, baking soda, and baking powder. Stir well.

3. Add shredded apples and carrots to flour mixture and stir until evenly distributed.

4. In small bowl, whisk together eggs, milk, and oil.

5. Create well in middle of dry ingredients; then pour liquid ingredients into well. Stir just until combined.

6. Bake 15–20 minutes until muffins are golden brown and thoroughly baked.

Yield: 12 muffins

## NUTRITION INFORMATION

Serving size: 1 muffin

Per serving: 180 calories, 6 g total fat, ½ g saturated fat, 30 mg cholesterol, 28 g carbohydrates, 3 g fiber, 13 g sugars, 4 g protein, and 170 mg sodium

CACFP: Serve with ¾ cup fluid milk and ¼ cup fruit (or 100 percent juice).

# Maple Granola Yogurt Parfait

Estimated preparation and cooking time: 2 days
(1 hour and 20 minutes the day before and 10 minutes the day of serving)

## INGREDIENTS

2 cups rolled oats

½ cup sunflower seeds

½ cup pumpkin seeds

2 tablespoons sesame seeds

½ teaspoon ground cinnamon

⅓ cup grade B maple syrup

2 tablespoons canola oil

¼ cup dried apricots (cut into small pieces)

¼ cup dried cranberries

2½ cups blueberries (fresh or frozen)

2½ cups sliced bananas

3 cups nonfat or low-fat vanilla yogurt

## PROCEDURE

### Day 1

1. Preheat oven to 275°F. Lightly grease rimmed baking sheet.

2. In large bowl, combine oats, seeds, and cinnamon.

3. Pour syrup and oil over mixture and stir until well combined.

4. Spread granola in prepared pan and bake for 1 hour and 10 minutes, stirring occasionally, until granola is golden brown. Note: granola will crisp as it cools.

5. Once granola is cool, stir in dried apricots and cranberries.

### Day 2

1. Slice bananas.

2. Prepare individual parfaits by layering 3 tablespoons yogurt, ¼ cup blueberries, 2 tablespoons granola, 3 tablespoons yogurt, ¼ cup sliced bananas, 2 tablespoons yogurt. Top with 3 tablespoons granola.

Yield: 10 servings

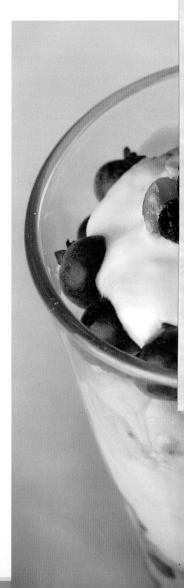

## NUTRITION INFORMATION

Serving size: ¹/₁₀ recipe

Per serving: 330 calories, 10 g total fat, 1½ g saturated fat, 5 mg cholesterol, 50 g carbohydrates, 5 g fiber, 29 g sugars, 11 g protein, and 60 mg sodium

CACFP: Serve with ¾ cup fluid milk to meet the breakfast requirements. (The Maple Granola Yogurt Parfait meets the snack food requirements as written.)

- Granola can be prepared a few days in advance and stored in an airtight container. Granola without dried fruit can be stored in the freezer for up to 3 months.

- Granola is a great source of whole grains, healthy fats, and fiber.

- Experiment with different types of dried fruits, such as cherries, apricots, raisins, blueberries, currants, and apples.

- Use other fresh or frozen fruits in the parfait, such as raspberries, blackberries, peaches, strawberries, apricots, and mangos.

- Grade B maple syrup has more intense maple flavor that can be tasted in baked goods.

- If your center allows nuts, try substituting slivered almonds for pumpkin seeds.

- Try adding granola to your pancake or waffle batters for a nutritional boost.

- Granola is a healthy cold breakfast cereal and is also great on top of applesauce.

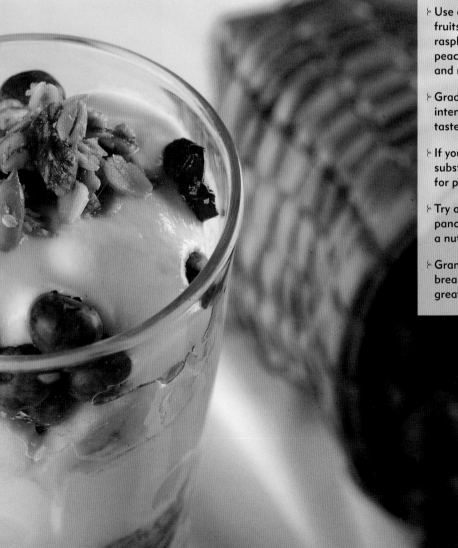

# Cinnamon-Oatmeal Pancakes

Estimated preparation and cooking time: 30 minutes

## INGREDIENTS

1 cup white whole wheat flour or whole wheat pastry flour

1 cup rolled oats

1½ tablespoons sugar

2 teaspoons baking powder

½ teaspoon baking soda

1 teaspoon ground cinnamon

1½ cups skim milk

1½ teaspoons vanilla extract

2 tablespoons canola oil

2 eggs

5 cups fresh fruit

Maple syrup (optional)

Nonstick cooking spray

## PROCEDURE

1. Place flour and oats in blender and blend until oats resemble coarse flour. Add remaining ingredients and purée until smooth.

2. Lightly spray nonstick skillet or electric griddle with nonstick cooking spray. Heat skillet on medium-high or electric griddle to 375°F.

3. Pour or scoop batter onto griddle, using approximately ⅛ cup (2 tablespoons) for each pancake. Cook until pancakes are puffed and browned on one side; flip and cook until browned on other side.

4. Serve with maple syrup or fresh fruit.

Yield: 12 servings

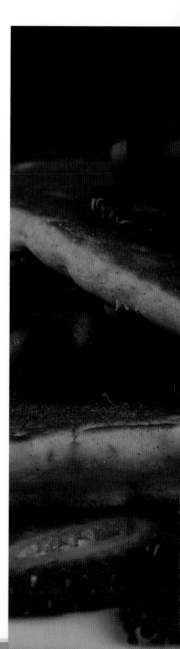

## NUTRITION INFORMATION

Serving size: 2 pancakes

Per serving (no fruit or syrup): 120 calories, 3½ g total fat, 30 mg cholesterol, 0 g saturated fat, 16 g carbohydrates, 2 g fiber, 4 g sugars, 5 g protein, and 140 mg sodium

CACFP: Serve 2 pancakes with ½ cup fruit and ¾ cup fluid milk.

Dietary fiber plays a positive role in overall digestive health, healthy body weight, and blood sugar regulation. Here are some tips for increasing dietary fiber:

- Look for products that list whole wheat or other whole grain flours as the first ingredient instead of enriched wheat flour.

- Replace all-purpose flour with white whole wheat or whole wheat pastry flour in your favorite recipes.

- Select products that contain at least 2½ grams of fiber per serving. Preschool-age children should consume 19–25 grams of dietary fiber daily.

- Add an extra serving of vegetables to your dinner plate.

- Add beans to your soup, salad, or pasta.

- Enjoy a salad at least once a day.

- Choose a fruit or vegetable with each snack.

- Add fruit to your breakfast cereal, or top whole grain pancakes with fresh fruit instead of maple syrup.

- Replace white pasta with whole grain pasta.

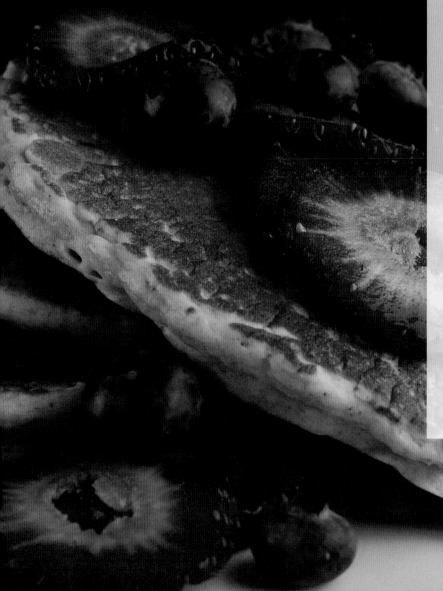

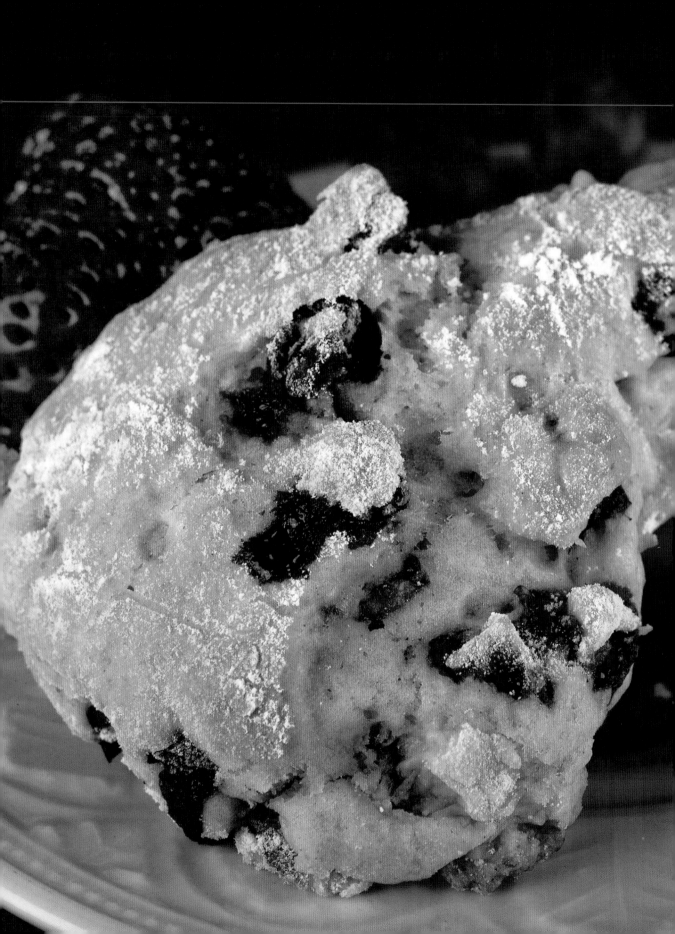

# Whole Grain Strawberry-Blueberry Scones

Estimated preparation and cooking time: 40 minutes

## INGREDIENTS

3 cups white whole wheat flour

4½ teaspoons baking powder

¼ teaspoon salt

1 teaspoon ground cinnamon

6 tablespoons sugar

1 cup frozen or fresh wild blueberries (organic preferred)

1 cup sliced frozen or fresh strawberries (organic preferred)

1 egg, beaten

6 tablespoons canola oil

¾ cup skim or soy milk

1 teaspoon vanilla extract

## PROCEDURE

1. **Preheat oven to 425°F.**

2. **In large mixing bowl, combine all dry ingredients; add blueberries and strawberries.**

3. **In smaller bowl, combine all wet ingredients and add to dry, stirring just until combined.**

4. **Separate dough into two portions. Place on countertop and press each portion into circle 1-inch thick.**

5. **Cut each circle into 8 wedges. Place each wedge on parchment-covered cookie sheet.**

6. **Bake 20–25 minutes or until golden brown.**

Yield: 16 scones

## NUTRITION INFORMATION

Serving size: 1 scone

Per serving: 170 calories, 6 g total fat, 0 g saturated fat, 10 mg cholesterol, 26 g carbohydrates, 3 g fiber, 7 g sugars, 4 g protein, and 160 mg sodium.

CACFP: Serve with ¾ cup fluid milk and ½ cup fruit, such as fresh berries. (Serve with ½ cup milk or fruit to meet snack requirements.)

⌁ **Scones originated in the British Isles hundreds of years ago and are traditionally made with butter and cream. This is a much healthier version that is just as delicious!**

⌁ **A delicious variation on this recipe is to use just one type of berry. Try 2 cups of sliced strawberries or blueberries instead of 1 cup of each.**

⌁ **Use organic fruits to avoid exposure to pesticides and other chemicals.**

# Whole Grain Scones with Raisins

Estimated preparation and cooking time: 35 minutes

## INGREDIENTS

3 cups white whole wheat flour

4½ teaspoons baking powder

¼ teaspoon salt

1 teaspoon ground cinnamon

6 tablespoons sugar

1 cup raisins (organic preferred)

1 egg, beaten

6 tablespoons canola oil

¾ cup skim or soy milk

1 teaspoon vanilla extract

## PROCEDURE

1. Preheat oven to 425°F.

2. In large mixing bowl, combine all dry ingredients; add raisins.

3. In smaller bowl, combine all wet ingredients and add to dry, stirring just until combined.

4. Separate dough into two portions. Place on countertop and press each portion into circle 1-inch thick.

5. Cut each circle into 8 wedges. Place each wedge on parchment-covered cookie sheet.

6. Bake 20–25 minutes or until golden brown.

Yield: 16 scones

## NUTRITION INFORMATION

Serving size: 1 scone

Per serving: 190 calories, 6 g total fat, 0 g saturated fat, 10 mg cholesterol, 31 g carbohydrates, 3 g fiber, 11 g sugars, 4 g protein, and 160 mg sodium.

CACFP: Serve with ¾ cup fluid milk and ½ cup fruit, such as fresh berries. (Serve with ½ cup milk or fruit to meet snack requirements.)

⸓ The recipe can be made with different types of dried, fresh, or frozen fruits.

⸓ Round scones can be made by rolling the dough to 1-inch thickness and cutting with the top of a drinking cup.

⸓ Use organic raisins to avoid exposure to pesticides and other chemicals.

# Whole Grain Cranberry-Orange Scones

Estimated preparation and cooking time: 40 minutes   (DAIRY FREE)

## INGREDIENTS

3 cups white whole wheat flour

4½ teaspoons baking powder

¼ teaspoon salt

6 tablespoons sugar

1 cup dried cranberries (organic preferred)

1 egg, beaten

6 tablespoons canola oil

¾ cup orange juice

Grated rind of 1 orange (organic preferred)

## PROCEDURE

1. Preheat oven to 425°F.
2. In large mixing bowl, combine all dry ingredients; add cranberries.
3. In smaller bowl, combine all wet ingredients and add to dry, stirring just until combined.
4. Separate dough into two portions. Place on countertop and press each portion into circle 1-inch thick.
5. Cut each circle into 8 wedges. Place each wedge on parchment-covered cookie sheet.
6. Bake 20–25 minutes or until golden brown.

Yield: 16 scones

## NUTRITION INFORMATION

Serving size: 1 scone

Per serving: 190 calories, 6 g total fat, 0 g saturated fat, 10 mg cholesterol, 30 g carbohydrates, 3 g fiber, 10 g sugars, 3 g protein, and 150 mg sodium

CACFP: Serve with ¾ cup fluid milk and ½ cup fruit, such as fresh berries. (Serve with ½ cup milk or fruit to meet snack requirements.)

⊱ These scones are perfect for children and adults who have allergies to dairy products.

⊱ Dried cherries can be substituted for cranberries in this recipe.

⊱ Use organic fruit to avoid exposure to pesticides and other chemicals. Organic dried cranberries are available online as well as at many grocery stores.

# Whole Grain Lemon-Poppy Scones

Estimated preparation and cooking time: 40 minutes

## INGREDIENTS

3 cups white whole wheat flour

4½ teaspoons baking powder

¼ teaspoon salt

1 teaspoon ground cinnamon

6 tablespoons sugar

2 tablespoons poppy seeds

1 egg, beaten

6 tablespoons canola oil

¾ cup skim or soy milk

Grated rind of 1 lemon (organic preferred)

## PROCEDURE

1. Preheat oven to 425°F.

2. In large mixing bowl, combine all dry ingredients, including poppy seeds.

3. In smaller bowl, combine all wet ingredients and add to dry, stirring just until combined.

4. Separate dough into two portions. Place on countertop and press each portion into circle 1-inch thick.

5. Cut each circle into 8 wedges. Place each wedge on parchment-covered cookie sheet.

6. Bake 20–25 minutes or until golden brown.

Yield: 16 scones

## NUTRITION INFORMATION

Serving size: 1 scone

Per serving: 170 calories, 6 g total fat, ½ g saturated fat, 10 mg cholesterol, 24 g carbohydrates, 3 g fiber, 5 g sugars, 4 g protein, and 160 mg sodium

CACFP: Serve with ¾ cup fluid milk and ½ cup fruit, such as fresh berries. (Serve with ½ cup milk or fruit to meet snack requirements.)

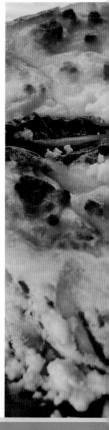

⨍ The origin of the word *scone* is not known. It could be Scottish, Dutch, German, or Gaelic.

⨍ In North America, the pronunciation of *scone* usually rhymes with *cone*. In England and Scotland, however, the word usually rhymes with *John*.

# Zucchini-Tomato Casserole

Estimated preparation and cooking time: 55 minutes

## INGREDIENTS

8 large eggs

½ cup skim milk

4 ounces feta cheese, crumbled

1½ cups shredded zucchini (about 1 large zucchini)

1 cup grape tomatoes, quartered

Nonstick cooking spray

## PROCEDURE

1. Preheat oven to 350°F. Lightly coat large pie pan or 12-inch square casserole dish with nonstick cooking spray.

2. In medium bowl, beat eggs and milk together until well combined.

3. Add shredded zucchini and crumbled feta to mixture. Gently stir to combine.

4. Pour mixture into pie pan. Gently top with quartered grape tomatoes.

5. Bake 40–45 minutes or until knife inserted into center of dish comes out clean.

6. For golden brown top, broil 1–2 minutes on medium. Watch constantly to avoid burning.

7. Allow to cool slightly before serving.

Yield: 10 servings

## NUTRITION INFORMATION

Serving size: ¹⁄₁₀ recipe

Per serving: 100 calories, 6 g total fat, 2½ g saturated fat, 155 mg cholesterol, 3 g carbohydrates, 0 g fiber, 3 g sugars, 7 g protein, and 190 mg sodium

CACFP: Serve with ¾ cup fluid milk, ¼ cup fruit (such as a small bunch of halved grapes), and ½ slice whole grain toast.

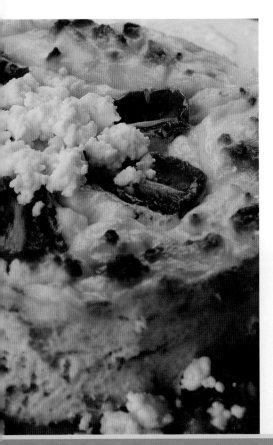

⸓ Eggs are one of the few foods that naturally contain vitamin D, the vitamin we get from the sun during the summer months.

⸓ How do you tell if an egg is uncooked or hard-boiled? If it easily spins, it's hard-boiled. If it wobbles, it's raw.

⸓ How do you tell if an egg is fresh? A fresh egg will sink when placed in a bowl of water, but an old egg will float because its air pocket has increased in size.

# SIX

―∽―

# LUNCH
# RECIPES

THERE IS SO MUCH TO BE LEARNED at lunchtime in a preschool setting! It is a time for children to develop fine-motor skills as they
serve themselves, to practice social skills, and to be adventurous and
try new foods. A teacher has many opportunities throughout the course of a
meal to teach through modeling—guiding the conversation, eating healthy
foods eagerly, and being enthusiastic when new foods are available to taste.
Daily opportunities for impromptu nutrition lessons abound when you talk
to children about the foods they eat at school and at home.

Lunchtime in preschool provides another opportunity to help children
develop healthy eating habits if the staff becomes committed to eliminating
menu offerings like peanut butter and jelly, chicken nuggets, and fish sticks,
which are commonly served as lunch for young children. This chapter contains recipes for lunches that feature nutritious ingredients, such as whole
grains, low-fat dairy, and lots of vegetables.

The Child and Adult Care Food Program (CACFP) requires four lunch
components for children ages three to five years:

1. ¾ cup fluid milk

2. A minimum of two different vegetables, fruit, or juice to equal ½ cup

3. ½ slice of bread (enriched or whole grain), ⅓ cup cold cereal
   (enriched or whole grain), ¼ cup hot cereal (enriched or whole
   grain), or ¼ cup cooked pasta or noodle products

4. 1½ ounces of cooked meat, poultry, or fish, 1½ ounces of cheese,
   ¾ large egg, ⅜ cup of cooked dried beans or peas, 3 tablespoons
   of peanut or other nut/seed butters, ¾ ounce of nuts or seeds, or
   6 ounces of yogurt.

The recipes in this chapter fulfill one to three of the CACFP lunch
components with a note in the nutrition information section that guides you
in easily meeting the remaining requirements.

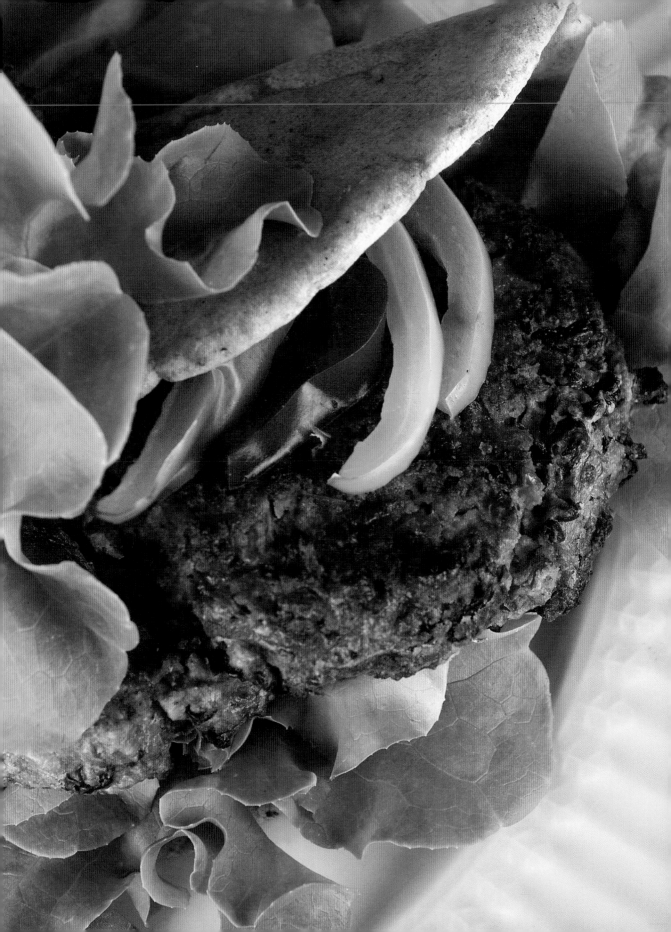

# Bell Pepper Veggie Burgers

Estimated preparation and cooking time: 35 minutes

## INGREDIENTS

1½ medium red bell peppers

1 tablespoon canola oil

4 eggs

2 cans (15 ounce) low-sodium black beans, drained and rinsed

1⅓ cups Italian bread crumbs

1 cup shredded cheddar cheese

Nonstick cooking spray

Ketchup

⋅ These burgers are a healthy vegetarian alternative to ground beef burgers—the beans add fiber and are low in fat.

⋅ Bell peppers are a good source of vitamins A, C, and B6 and potassium.

⋅ Red bell peppers are green bell peppers that have been allowed to ripen.

⋅ Bell peppers are related to hot peppers but contain a recessive gene that lacks spiciness. They are from the same family as eggplant and tomatoes.

⋅ Paprika is made by grinding dried red bell peppers.

## PROCEDURE

1. Preheat oven to broil. Spray baking sheet generously with nonstick cooking spray.

2. Wash, destem, and deseed bell peppers. Cut into ¼-inch pieces.

3. Place vegetable oil in skillet. Heat on medium. When oil is hot, add peppers. Sauté until tender.

4. In small bowl, lightly beat eggs with fork or whisk.

5. Place beans in large bowl and mash well with potato masher or large fork.

6. Add peppers, bread crumbs, lightly beaten eggs, and cheese to mashed beans. Stir until evenly combined.

7. Form burger mixture into 10 patties and place on baking sheet. Set in oven 4–6 inches from flame. Broil 5 minutes, flip burgers, and broil 5–6 minutes more. Watch closely to prevent burning.

8. When burgers are done, cool slightly before placing in halved or quartered pita pockets. Serve family-style with low-sodium ketchup and enjoy!

9. (Alternative cooking method: Cook on stovetop on medium-high 4–5 minutes per side, or to internal temperature of 160°F, in skillet coated with vegetable oil.)

Yield: 10 servings

## NUTRITION INFORMATION

Serving size: 1 burger

Per serving: 170 calories, 6 g total fat, 2 g saturated fat, 80 mg cholesterol, 22 g carbohydrates, 4 g fiber, 3 g sugars, 10 g protein, and 510 mg sodium

CACFP: Serve with ¼ large or ½ small whole wheat pita bread, ¾ cup fluid milk, and 2 vegetables or 1 fruit and 1 vegetable to total ½ cup.

# Boston Baked Bean Cups

Estimated preparation and cooking time: 1 hour and 15 minutes

## INGREDIENTS

### BOSTON BAKED BEAN FILLING

1 tablespoon canola oil

¼ cup onion, minced

2 tablespoons ketchup

2 tablespoons dark molasses

1 teaspoon dry ground mustard

½ tablespoon cider vinegar

2 cans (15-ounce) low-sodium pinto beans, drained and rinsed

A good pinch each of ground cloves, ginger, black pepper, garlic powder

### CORN MUFFIN CRUST

1 cup white whole wheat flour

10 tablespoons cornmeal

2 teaspoons sugar

2½ teaspoons baking powder

¼ teaspoon salt

1 egg

2 tablespoons canola oil

⅔ cup skim milk

1½ cups reduced-fat cheddar cheese, shredded

Nonstick cooking spray

## PROCEDURE

1. In large sauce pan, sauté onion in 1 tablespoon canola oil on medium-high until soft and translucent.

2. Add ketchup, molasses, mustard, vinegar, beans, and spices. Mix together and bring to boil. Reduce heat and cook 15–20 minutes or until sauce has thickened and reduced.

3. While bean mixture is cooking, preheat oven to 375°F. Coat 12-cup muffin pan with nonstick cooking spray.

4. Combine flour, cornmeal, sugar, baking powder, and salt in medium bowl.

5. In another small bowl, lightly beat egg. Add 2 tablespoons oil and milk; mix well with beaten egg.

6. Combine dry and wet ingredients; stir until dry ingredients are moistened.

7. Divide batter between muffin cups. Using lightly oiled spoon, gently spread batter up sides of muffin cups to form cups.

8. When bean filling is cooked, spoon it into dough cups, dividing beans evenly.

9. Bake 15 minutes.

10. Remove from oven and top beans with shredded cheese—2 tablespoons per cup.

11. Bake 5–10 minutes or until cheese is melted and crusts are brown.

12. Let stand 10 minutes before serving. Use knife to loosen bean cups from muffin tin.

Yield: 12 bean cups

## NUTRITION INFORMATION

Serving size: 1 baked bean cup

Per serving: 190 calories, 7 g total fat, 2 g saturated fat, 10 mg cholesterol, 24 g carbohydrates, 4 g fiber, 3 g sugars, 8 g protein, and 280 mg sodium

CACFP: Serve with ¾ cup fluid milk and 2 vegetables or 1 fruit and 1 vegetable to total ½ cup.

꙳ For most of the world, the word *corn* means any kind of grain. In many countries, people would say the crust in this recipe is made from *maize*.

꙳ Maize is an important part of traditional diets in many parts of the world, including Central and South America, Africa, and parts of Asia. In Europe and North America, more of it is eaten by livestock than by humans.

꙳ The baked bean filling in this recipe is an easy way to enjoy the flavors of traditional Boston Baked Beans. Authentic baked bean recipes require several hours of cooking time.

꙳ The early settlers in Massachusetts learned to make baked beans from American Indians, who sweetened their beans with maple syrup.

꙳ The baked bean filling can be served on its own as a meat alternative—serve ½ cup per child for lunch.

# Chili Bean Cups

Estimated preparation and cooking time: 1 hour and 15 minutes

## INGREDIENTS

### CHILI BEAN FILLING

¾ cup tomato sauce

¾ teaspoon chili powder

¼ teaspoon cumin

⅛ teaspoon salt

2 cans (15-ounce) low-sodium pinto beans, drained and rinsed

### CORN MUFFIN CRUST

1 cup white whole wheat flour

10 tablespoons cornmeal

2 teaspoons sugar

2½ teaspoons baking powder

¼ teaspoon salt

1 egg

2 tablespoons canola oil

⅔ cup skim milk

1½ cups reduced-fat cheddar cheese, shredded

Nonstick cooking spray

## PROCEDURE

1. In large saucepan, combine tomato sauce, chili powder, cumin, salt, and pinto beans. Mix well.

2. Bring mixture to boil, reduce heat, cook 15–20 minutes or until sauce has thickened and reduced.

3. While bean mixture cooks, preheat oven to 375°F. Coat 12-cup muffin pan with nonstick cooking spray.

4. Combine flour, cornmeal, sugar, baking powder, and salt in medium bowl.

5. In small bowl, lightly beat egg. Add 2 tablespoons oil and milk; mix well.

6. Combine dry and wet ingredients; stir until dry ingredients are moistened.

7. Divide batter between muffin cups. Using oiled spoon, gently spread batter up sides of muffin cups to form cups.

8. When chili bean filling is cooked, spoon into dough cups, dividing beans evenly.

9. Bake 15 minutes.

10. Remove from oven and top beans with shredded cheese—2 tablespoons per bean cup.

11. Bake 5–10 minutes or until cheese is melted and crusts are brown.

12. Let stand 10 minutes before serving. Use knife to loosen bean cups from muffin tin.

Yield: 12 bean cups

## NUTRITION INFORMATION

Serving size: 1 chili bean cup

Per serving: 160 calories, 5 g total fat, 2 g saturated fat, 25 mg cholesterol, 22 g carbohydrates, 4 g fiber, 2 g sugars, 9 g protein, and 360 mg sodium

CACFP: Serve with ¾ cup fluid milk and 2 vegetables or 1 fruit and 1 vegetable to total ½ cup.

⊱ Cornmeal is a minimally processed whole grain containing dietary fiber, nutrients, and minerals.

⊱ **The chili bean filling is a simplified vegetarian version of a favorite American dish. Traditionally, chili is made with meat, not beans.**

⊱ Contrary to popular belief, chili originated in the United States, not Mexico. Many people believe that chili was first made and eaten by cowboys on cattle drives in the early 1800s. Others trace its origins to the city of San Antonio, Texas, where it was made by immigrants from the Canary Islands.

⊱ The chili bean filling can be served on its own as a meat alternative—serve ½ cup per child for lunch.

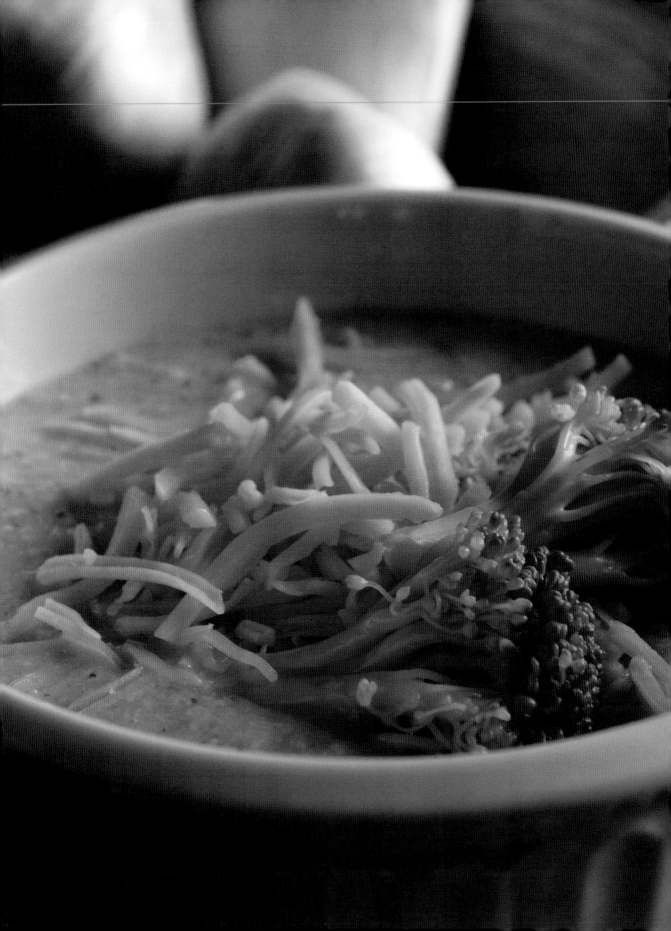

# Broccoli-Cheddar Soup

Estimated preparation and cooking time: 35 minutes

## INGREDIENTS

4 cups chopped broccoli

½ cup diced onion

1 clove garlic, pressed or minced

1 tablespoon canola oil

3½ cups water or vegetable stock

3 cups canellini beans (2 15-ounce cans, drained and rinsed)

5 ounces reduced-fat sharp cheddar cheese, shredded

⅛ teaspoon salt

⅛ teaspoon ground black pepper

## PROCEDURE

1. In large stockpot, heat canola oil on medium-high. Add onion and garlic; sauté until onion is soft and translucent.

2. Add water or vegetable stock and bring to boil. Add broccoli; cook until tender, about 8–10 minutes, depending on size of broccoli pieces.

3. Stir in beans, salt, and pepper; continue cooking until beans are heated through.

4. Remove pot from heat and stir in cheese. Using either immersion blender or food processor, purée soup until smooth. (If using food processor, you may need to work in two or more batches.)

5. If needed, reheat gently and serve.

Yield: 10 servings

⸙ This is a healthy version of a soup that is a popular choice in many restaurants. Our version is lower in fat and sodium and higher in fiber.

⸙ Broccoli is a cruciferous vegetable (like cauliflower and kale) and is an excellent source of vitamins A, C, and K, calcium, and folate, as well as several other phytonutrients. It is believed to help protect against a variety of cancers as well as heart disease and is widely considered a superfood because of its high nutritional value.

⸙ The word *broccoli* comes from the Italian word for "branch" or "arm."

⸙ Broccoli was first brought to North America by Italian immigrants during colonial times. Thomas Jefferson grew broccoli at Monticello.

## NUTRITION INFORMATION

Serving size: ¹/₁₀ recipe

Per serving: 130 calories, 5 g total fat, 2 g saturated fat, 10 mg cholesterol, 14 g carbohydrates, 4 g fiber, 2 g sugars, 8 g protein, and 190 mg sodium

CACFP: Serve with ¾ cup fluid milk, ¼ cup fruit or vegetable, and ½ slice whole grain bread.

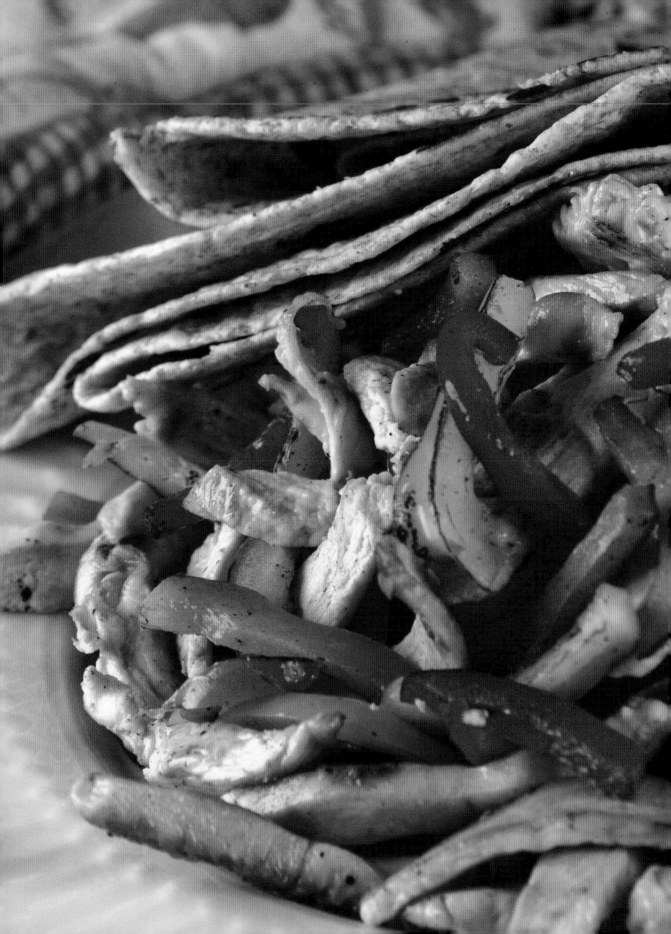

# Chicken Fajitas

Estimated preparation and cooking time: 1–3 hours in advance and 30 minutes immediately before serving

## INGREDIENTS

1½ pounds chicken breast, boneless, skinless

Juice from 2 limes

⅛ teaspoon ground black pepper

2 teaspoons ground cumin

1½ tablespoons brown sugar

1 teaspoon chili powder

3 teaspoons canola oil, divided into 1 teaspoon and 2 teaspoons

1¼ pound red or green bell peppers, sliced

1 large onion, chopped or sliced

1 can (15-ounce) black beans, low-sodium, drained and rinsed

10 whole wheat tortillas

⸖ Warming the tortillas makes them more flexible and easier to work with. Wrap them in a damp paper towel and microwave for 30–60 seconds.

⸖ Fajitas were originally made from a tough cut of beef called *skirt steak*. The Spanish word *faja*, which means "belt," was also used to refer to the skirt steak, and is the root of the word *fajita*. Today, any kind of meat that is served in a wheat flour tortilla can be called a fajita.

⸖ Boneless, skinless chicken breast is a good source of lean protein. It's high in vitamin B6, niacin, and selenium, and low in saturated fat.

⸖ There are more chickens in the world than there are humans.

## PROCEDURE

1. Cut chicken breasts into thin strips and place in bowl. Squeeze lime juice onto chicken strips and refrigerate 1–3 hours.

2. In small bowl, combine black pepper, cumin, brown sugar, and chili powder; mix to create dry rub.

3. Evenly coat chicken strips with dry rub.

4. Heat 1 teaspoon oil in large skillet on medium heat. Add chicken to skillet and stir-fry on medium-low until chicken is cooked through, about 10 minutes (or an internal temperature of 165°F is reached).

5. Heat remaining 2 teaspoons oil in separate skillet on medium heat and stir-fry peppers and onion until softened.

6. Place black beans in glass bowl and warm in microwave.

7. Assemble fajitas by dividing chicken, onion, and pepper mixture and black beans evenly among tortillas. Place fillings in center of each tortilla, bring bottom edge of tortilla over filling, tuck in sides, and roll up.

Yield: 10 servings

## NUTRITION INFORMATION

Serving size: 1 filled tortilla

Per serving: 280 calories, 5 g total fat, 0 g saturated fat, 40 mg cholesterol, 35 g carbohydrates, 5 g fiber, 5 g sugars, 22 g protein, and 310 mg sodium

CACFP: Serve with ¾ cup fluid milk.

# Hummus & Veggie Bar

Estimated preparation and cooking time: 45 minutes

## INGREDIENTS

2 cans (15-ounce) reduced-sodium chickpeas, drained and rinsed

3 tablespoons tahini

1 tablespoon lemon juice

¼–½ teaspoon garlic powder

Salt to taste

1 red bell pepper

10 whole wheat tortillas

1½ cups shredded reduced fat cheddar cheese

2½ cups shredded raw carrots

2½ cups shredded raw beets

2½ cups chopped cucumbers

## PROCEDURE

1. Preheat oven to broil.

2. Combine chickpeas, tahini, lemon juice, garlic powder, and salt in food processor. Process until mixture is smooth.

3. Place whole pepper in baking pan on highest oven rack under broiler and watch it carefully; when black scorched spots begin to appear, remove pepper from oven and turn over, using tongs. Return to oven and repeat until entire pepper is covered with scorched spots.

4. Place scorched pepper in glass or metal bowl and cover tightly with plastic wrap. Let sit for 15 minutes (this makes removing skin easy).

5. Once pepper is cool enough to handle, remove stem, seeds, and skin.

6. Add roasted pepper to chickpea mixture. Process until pepper is chopped and distributed evenly throughout mixture.

7. Top whole wheat tortillas with hummus, cheese, and vegetables.

Yield: 10 servings

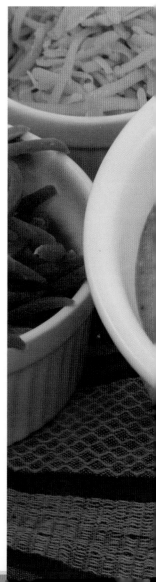

## NUTRITION INFORMATION

Serving size: 1 tortilla, ¼ cup hummus, 2 tablespoons cheese

Per serving: 260 calories, 10 g total fat, 2½ g saturated fat, 10 mg cholesterol, 30 g carbohydrates, 4 g fiber, 3 g sugars, 12 g protein, and 360 mg sodium

CACFP: 1 tortilla topped with ¼ cup hummus, 2 tablespoons cheese, and ¼ cup two different vegetables meets the lunch requirements when served with ¾ cup fluid milk.

- Set up a hummus bar and let children serve themselves; they can construct their own wraps, topping tortillas, hummus, and cheese with the vegetables of their choice.

- Hummus is also good served as a dip for vegetables or whole wheat pita bread—it's higher in fiber and lower in fat than sour cream-based dips.

- Chickpeas are high in fiber, protein, folate, and iron.

- Sweet and crunchy raw beets are popular with young children. They make a healthy topping for sandwiches and salads.

- Beets are loaded with nutrients: fiber, vitamin C, folate, magnesium, and iron. The dark pigment is a phytonutrient believed to fight cancer.

- Don't be alarmed if eating beets causes urine and feces to take on a pink tinge. Some people don't digest the pigment well; it simply passes through the body and is excreted.

# Macaroni, Squash, & Cheese

Estimated preparation and cooking time: 1 hour and 15 minutes

## INGREDIENTS

2½ cups cooked butternut squash

1 medium bunch Swiss chard
(5 cups chopped)

½ pound whole wheat pasta

1 tablespoon canola oil

1 tablespoon flour

1 cup skim milk

1 cup shredded reduced-fat sharp
cheddar cheese

½ teaspoon garlic powder

¼ cup bread crumbs

¼ cup Parmesan cheese

Nonstick cooking spray

## PROCEDURE

1. Preheat oven to 400°F. Fill baking dish with 1 inch of water.

2. Cut butternut squash in half from top to bottom. Do not scoop out seeds. Place squash cut-side down in baking dish with water; bake 30–40 minutes or until flesh is soft.

3. Allow squash to cool thoroughly. Scoop out seeds and discard them. Scoop out 2½ cups cooked squash.

4. Turn oven to 425°F.

5. Bring pot of water to boil.

6. Wash Swiss chard, remove stems, and cut leaves into small, ⅓–½-inch pieces.

7. When water boils, add pasta and cook until al dente (9 minutes), stirring occasionally.

8. Add cut-up Swiss chard to pot and cook with pasta for 1 minute.

9. Drain pasta and Swiss chard in colander.

10. Heat same pot on medium, add oil, then flour, and cook, stirring constantly, until mixture resembles thick paste but has not browned (1 to 2 minutes).

11. Add milk, stirring constantly until mixture starts to thicken (about 3 minutes).

12. Combine squash, cheese, and garlic powder into thickened mixture, stirring until cheese melts.

13. Add drained pasta and Swiss chard to cheese sauce and stir to combine.

14. Lightly coat 9 x 13-inch baking pan with nonstick cooking spray. Spread pasta mixture in pan.

15. Mix bread crumbs and Parmesan together; sprinkle evenly over pasta mixture. Bake in 400°F oven for 10 minutes.

Yield: 10 servings

## NUTRITION INFORMATION

Serving size: 1/10 of recipe

Per serving: 190 calories, 5 g total fat, 2½ g saturated fat, 10 mg cholesterol, 28 g carbohydrates, 4 g fiber, 2 g sugars, 9 g protein, and 200 mg sodium

CACFP: Serve with ¾ cup fluid milk and 1½ ounces meat, or 6 ounces yogurt, or ¾ ounce nuts or seeds, or ⅜ cup beans.

- Spinach can be substituted for Swiss chard in this recipe.

- *Al dente* refers to the texture of cooked pasta. It means "to the tooth": the pasta offers some resistance when you bite into it. It is not soft or mushy.

- Swiss chard is optional—if you leave it out, serve with ¼ cup fruit or another vegetable to meet CACFP lunch requirements.

- Chard is a member of the beet family, but we eat only the leaves, not the root. Other related vegetables include mustard greens, kale, and spinach.

- Like many dark leafy greens, chard is a good source of vitamins A, C, E, and K, as well as folic acid, zinc, calcium, iron, magnesium, and potassium.

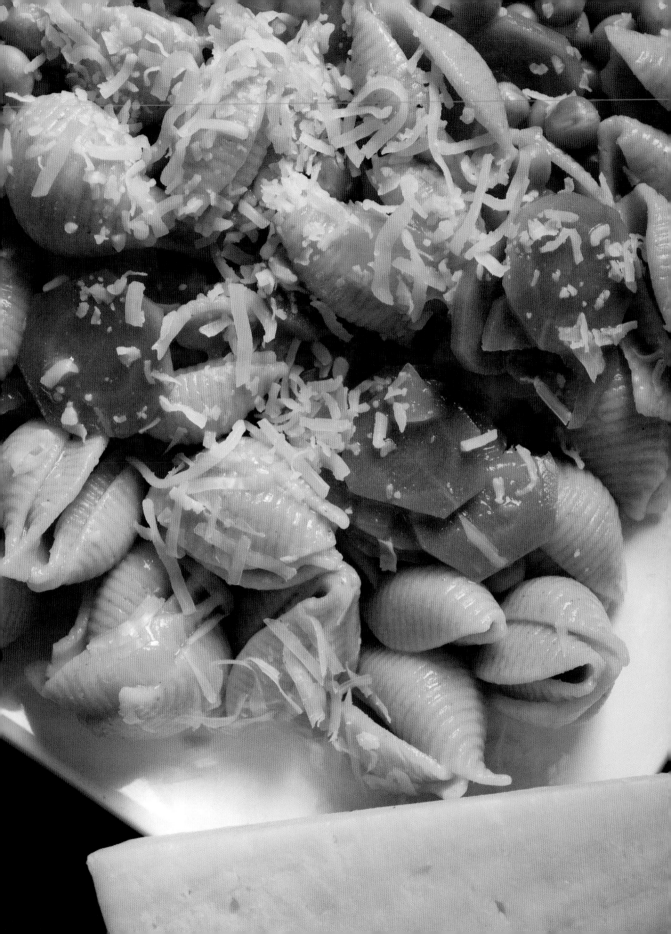

# Pasta with Peas & Carrots

Estimated preparation and cooking time: 40 minutes

## INGREDIENTS

10 ounces whole wheat pasta

2 teaspoons canola oil

1 small onion, diced

2½ cups sliced carrots

2½ cups frozen peas

2 cups vegetable broth

1 teaspoon butter

All-purpose flour

Salt and pepper to taste

1 cup grated Parmesan cheese

⸎ Steaming the whole carrots beforehand makes it easier for children to slice them.

⸎ Try making this dish with different vegetables—for example, zucchini, summer squash and broccoli.

⸎ Peas are legumes and high in fiber, vitamins A, C, and K, thiamine, niacin, folate, and iron. They're also a good source of protein—dried split peas can be cooked and eaten as an alternative to meat.

⸎ Peas have been used as a food for a long time. Archaeologists have found them in 4,000-year-old Egyptian tombs!

⸎ Peas were Thomas Jefferson's favorite vegetable. He grew fifteen different varieties.

⸎ You've probably heard the nursery rhyme "Pease Porridge Hot." Pease porridge was a staple food in Europe during the middle ages. Made from peas, it resembled a thick pea soup.

## PROCEDURE

1. Cook pasta according to package directions. Drain.

2. Heat canola oil in large pot on medium-high. Add diced onion and sauté until translucent.

3. Add carrots to pan and sauté until soft.

4. Add frozen peas and vegetable broth to pan and bring to boil.

5. While broth heats, cut butter into two pieces and roll both in all-purpose flour, coating each piece well.

6. When broth comes to a boil, add flour-coated butter; stir until broth thickens. Add salt and pepper.

7. Add pasta to sauce and mix well. Add Parmesan and mix well.

8. Cool slightly and serve.

Yield: 10 servings

## NUTRITION INFORMATION

Serving size: ¹⁄₁₀ recipe

Per serving: 200 calories, 5 g total fat, 2 g saturated fat, 10 mg cholesterol, 30 g carbohydrates, 5 g fiber, 4 g sugars, 11 g protein, and 280 mg sodium

CACFP: Serve with ¾ cup fluid milk and 1½ ounces cheese or lean meat, or ⅜ cup beans, or ¾ of a large egg, or ¾ ounce nuts or seeds, or 6 ounces yogurt.

# Whole Grain Veggie Pizza

Est. prep /cooking time: 2 days (1 hr., 45 min. day before; 40 min. day of serving).

## INGREDIENTS

1½ cups white whole wheat flour

1½ cups enriched all-purpose flour

1 teaspoon salt

1½ teaspoons yeast

1 cup very warm water

1 cup tomato sauce, low-sodium

4½ cups shredded part-skim mozzarella cheese

1½ cups diced bell peppers

1½ cups chopped broccoli

Nonstick cooking spray

## PROCEDURE

1. Place flour, salt, and yeast in large bowl. Gradually add water, mixing until dough forms ball. (You may need to add more water, depending on humidity.)

2. Flour clean tabletop or large cutting board and place dough on it. Knead dough, mixing in rest of flour, for 5–10 minutes or until dough is smooth and elastic. (You may need to add another tablespoon or two of water or flour.)

3. Lightly coat large bowl with nonstick cooking spray and place the dough in bowl, turning dough so all surfaces are lightly oiled. Cover bowl with plastic wrap. Allow dough to rise 1½ –3 hours at room temperature.

4. If dough will not be used right away, place in large plastic ziplock bag and put in refrigerator. Refrigerate dough 4–36 hours (bring it to room temperature again before using).

5. Preheat oven to 450°F; coat two large baking sheets with nonstick cooking spray.

6. Punch down dough and place on lightly floured surface. Divide dough into 2 round balls and flour lightly. Working with one ball of dough at a time, roll or press the dough evenly into 12-inch circle; place carefully on baking sheet.

7. Spread each pizza with ½ cup tomato sauce. Sprinkle mozzarella evenly over sauce.

8. Distribute vegetable toppings evenly over pizzas.

9. Bake 10–13 minutes or until crust is golden and cheese is melted. Cool slightly and cut each pizza into 12 slices.

Yield: 12 servings

## NUTRITION INFORMATION

Serving size: 2 slices

Per serving: 260 calories, 9 g total fat, 5 g saturated fat, 25 mg cholesterol, 34 g carbohydrates, 3 g fiber, 3 g sugars, 16 g protein, and 430 mg sodium

CACFP: Serve 2 slices with ¼ cup fruit and ¾ cup fluid milk per child.

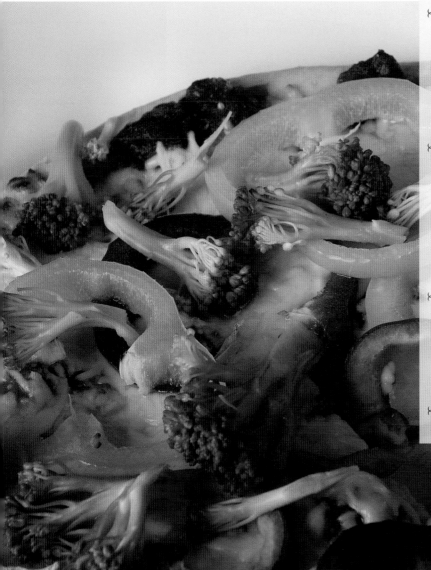

- If you find that the dough keeps springing back when you try to roll it out, let it rest for a minute or two—the dough will "relax" and be easier to roll.

- Children enjoy kneading and rolling pizza dough and helping to add toppings. They can also make their own pizzas—give them each a portion of dough and let them choose what to put on it.

- Many vegetables can be used as pizza toppings—be adventurous! Some other possibilities include:
  - artichoke hearts
  - mushrooms
  - zucchini or summer squash
  - eggplant
  - black beans

- Pizza is enjoyed all over the world—here are some toppings you might find in other countries:
  - ginger, mutton, and tofu (India)
  - eel and octopus (Japan)
  - fish (Russia)
  - bacon (France)
  - peas (Brazil)
  - coconut (Costa Rica)

- Although we tend to think of pizza as junk food, it doesn't have to be. Making your own whole wheat crust and topping it with part-skim mozzarella and lots of vegetables turns pizza into a nutritious meal.

- In the United States, October is National Pizza Month.

# Sweet Potato & Black Bean Quesadillas

Estimated preparation and cooking time: 30 minutes. Note: sweet potatoes are cooked in advance

## INGREDIENTS

2–3 large sweet potatoes (enough to yield 3 cups of mashed sweet potato), baked or microwaved until soft

6 nine-inch whole wheat tortillas

2¼ cups shredded reduced-fat cheddar cheese

1½ cans (15-ounce) low-sodium black beans

⅜ teaspoon garlic powder

¾ teaspoon ground cumin

Nonstick cooking spray

## PROCEDURE

1. Preheat oven to 350°F. Lightly coat baking sheets with nonstick cooking spray.

2. Place 3 tortillas on baking sheets. Spread ¾ cup shredded cheese over each tortilla.

3. Drain and rinse black beans. Evenly distribute ¾ cup beans over each cheese-topped tortilla.

4. Sprinkle ⅛ teaspoon garlic powder and ¼ teaspoon cumin over beans.

5. Split cooked sweet potatoes and scoop flesh from skins. Place flesh in bowl and mash. Measure out 3 cups.

6. Spread 1 cup mashed sweet potato on each remaining tortilla. Carefully turn these tortillas over atop cheese and bean tortillas; press down gently.

7. Lightly mist tops with nonstick cooking spray.

8. Bake for 20 minutes or until tortillas begin to turn golden.

9. Cool slightly, cut into quarters, and serve.

Yield: 12 servings

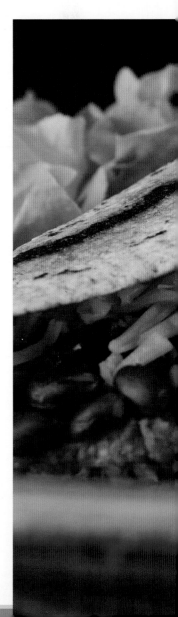

## NUTRITION INFORMATION

Serving size: ¼ of one quesadilla

Per serving: 200 calories, 6 g total fat, 2½ g saturated fat, 15 mg cholesterol, 30 g carbohydrates, 5 g fiber, 5 g sugars, 10 g protein, and 370 mg sodium

CACFP: Serve with ¾ cup fluid milk and ¼ cup fruit, such as peaches, quartered grapes, or berries.

⸙ Serve with reduced-fat sour cream and/or salsa, if desired.

⸙ Substitute pinto beans for black beans and try different types of cheeses, such as Monterey Jack.

⸙ Despite their sweet flavor, sweet potatoes are highly nutritious. They contain vitamins A, B6, and C, along with fiber, potassium, and iron, as well other antioxidant compounds.

⸙ In the United States, the moist orange-fleshed vegetables that many people call *yams* are actually sweet potatoes. True yams, which can grow to weigh 100 pounds, are related to lilies and grow in Africa and South America.

⸙ People have been eating sweet potatoes for at least 10,000 years, but they weren't known to Europeans until Columbus brought them back from the New World.

⸙ Black beans are another food loaded with nutrients, including fiber, iron, protein, folate, and antioxidants. They're economical, too—beans are a low-cost substitute for meat.

⸙ Many cultures around the world—African, Asian, South American, Indonesian, and Caribbean—consider beans an important staple food.

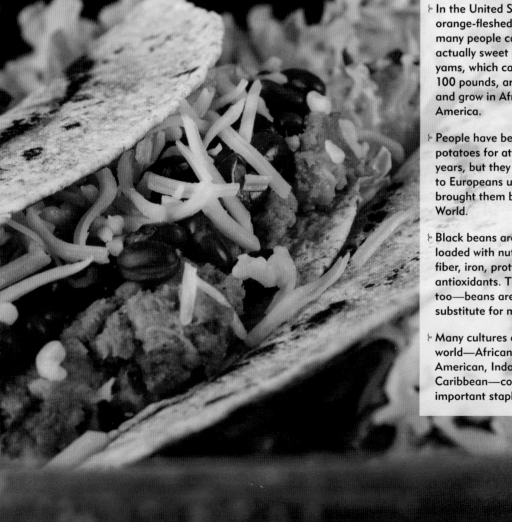

# Vegetable Lasagna

Estimated preparation and cooking time: 1 hour and 45 minutes

## INGREDIENTS

8 whole wheat lasagna noodles

1 tablespoon olive or canola oil

1 cup shredded or diced zucchini (about 1 small zucchini)

1 cup chopped broccoli

½ cup diced carrots

½ cup diced onion

2 cups nonfat cottage cheese

1 egg, beaten

Pinch of garlic powder

¼ teaspoon dried basil or 2 tablespoons chopped fresh basil

2 cups reduced-sodium spaghetti sauce

2 cups mozzarella cheese

¼ cup grated Parmesan cheese

Nonstick cooking spray

## PROCEDURE

1.  Lightly spray 8 x 8-inch baking pan with nonstick cooking spray.

2.  Cook lasagna noodles according to package directions.

3.  Preheat oven to 375°F.

4.  Heat oil in large skillet. Add zucchini, broccoli, carrots, and onion. Sauté until tender (about 15–20 minutes, depending on size of pieces). Set aside.

5.  Combine cottage cheese, beaten egg, garlic powder, and basil in small bowl; mix well.

6.  Spread ½ cup spaghetti sauce over bottom of pan. Build lasagna in layers as follows:

    a.  Place 4 noodles cut to fit pan on top of sauce, overlapping long edges.

    b.  Spread half of cottage cheese mixture evenly.

    c.  Spread half of sautéed vegetables over cottage cheese mixture.

    d.  Sprinkle half of mozzarella cheese evenly over vegetables.

    e.  Cover mozzarella with ¾ cup spaghetti sauce.

    f.  Place another 4 noodles on top of sauce.

    g.  Spread remaining cottage cheese mixture evenly over noodles.

    h.  Spread remaining vegetables evenly over cottage cheese mixture.

    i.  Spread remaining mozzarella over vegetables.

    j.  Lay one more layer of noodles.

    k.  Spread remaining sauce over noodles.

7.  Bake at 375°F 45–50 minutes. Add Parmesan cheese evenly over top and bake for 5 more minutes. Let sit for 10 minutes before serving.

Yield: 10 servings

## NUTRITION INFORMATION

Serving size: 1/10 recipe

Per serving: 230 calories, 9 g total fat, 4 g saturated fat, 40 mg cholesterol, 24 g carbohydrates, 3 g fiber, 6 g sugars, 14 g protein, and 280 mg sodium

CACFP: Serve with ¾ cup fluid milk and ¼ cup fruit, such as diced melon, apples, or pears.

⋋ Nonfat cottage cheese is a healthy alternative to the ricotta that is traditionally used in lasagna recipes—it's lower in calories and saturated fat.

⋋ Cottage cheese is the common name for the "curds and whey" that Miss Muffet ate in the nursery rhyme. It's called *cottage cheese* because it was easily made at home (in one's cottage).

⋋ It takes 100 pounds of milk to make 15 pounds of cottage cheese.

⋋ Most pasta is made from wheat, but it can also be made from other grains, such as buckwheat, rice, quinoa, even beans and vegetables.

⋋ Tomato sauce is rich in the antioxidant lycopene—cooking tomatoes for sauce actually makes it easier for our bodies to absorb lycopene.

⋋ The tomato is scientifically considered to be a fruit, but in 1893, the United States Supreme Court ruled that the tomato is a vegetable so it could be taxed.

———

# SEVEN

# SNACK
# RECIPES

Preschoolers need snacks. Their stomachs are too small to hold enough food to get them through the long stretch between meals. Children need to eat every two to three hours to gain enough energy to keep going and to obtain all the nutrients they need to stay healthy. Healthy snacking makes it easier for them to get the recommended 2½ to 3 cups of fruits and vegetables that many children otherwise lack. In child care settings, snacktime is also an important opportunity for social interaction. It also provides teachers chances to be good role models for healthy eating habits.

In American food culture, snacks usually mean chips, cookies, punch, and soda. At best, we may think of cheese and crackers as potential snack items. Snacking is a regular activity in young children's lives and, in fact, is required by child care licensing agencies. So, it is important that we take snacks seriously. In fact, they make up about 25 percent of the average preschool child's total caloric intake. Therefore we suggest thinking of snacks as mini meals.

The CACFP requires two snack components out of the following four for children ages three to five years:

1. ¾ cup fluid milk

2. ½ cup vegetables, fruit, or juice

3. ½ slice bread (enriched or whole grain), ⅓ cup cold cereal (enriched or whole grain), ¼ cup hot cereal (enriched or whole grain), or ¼ cup cooked pasta or noodle products

4. ½ ounce meat, cheese, or alternative protein, ½ egg, 2 ounces yogurt, ⅛ cup beans, or 1 tablespoon nut butter

Our recipes fulfill one to two of the CACFP snack components with a note in the nutrition information section that guides you in easily meeting the remaining requirements.

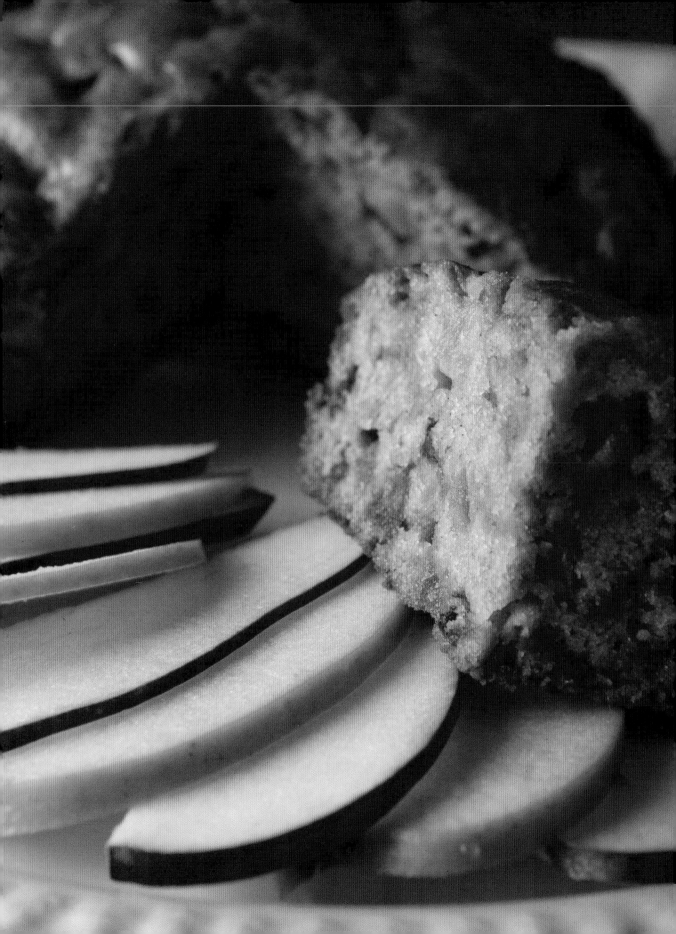

# Apple Snack Cake

Estimated preparation and cooking time: 50 minutes

## INGREDIENTS

5 cups unpeeled, cored apples

¾ cup sugar

⅓ cup canola oil

2 eggs, lightly beaten

1½ teaspoons vanilla extract

1½ cups white whole wheat flour
   or whole wheat pastry flour

1¼ teaspoons baking soda

1½ teaspoons ground cinnamon

Nonstick cooking spray

## PROCEDURE

1. Preheat oven to 350°F. Lightly spray 9 x 13-inch baking pan with nonstick cooking spray.

2. Chop unpeeled apples into small pieces and combine with sugar in large bowl. Stir well until evenly combined; set aside.

3. Combine oil, eggs, and vanilla in small mixing bowl.

4. In another large mixing bowl, combine flour, baking soda, and cinnamon. Stir until evenly combined.

5. Combine egg and flour mixtures. Stir until evenly combined.

6. Add combined mixtures slowly to apples. Stir until well combined.

7. Spread mixture evenly in prepared baking pan.

8. Bake 25–30 minutes or until cake tests done. Cool before serving.

Yield: 10 servings

## NUTRITION INFORMATION

Serving size: ¹⁄₁₀ recipe

Per serving: 250 calories, 9 g total fat, 1 g saturated fat, 35 mg cholesterol, 170 mg sodium, 39 g carbohydrates, 4 g fiber, 22 g sugar, 4 g protein

CACFP: ¹⁄₁₀ recipe meets the snack requirement.

ꙮ This is a great recipe to use during apple season, when apples are the most delicious and the least expensive. In the United States, apples are in season from late summer through early winter.

ꙮ Different varieties of apples have different flavors. Some apples are very sweet, while others are quite tart.

ꙮ Eating whole apples is much healthier than drinking apple juice. Whole apples have more fiber and phytonutrients (cancer-preventing agents). In fact, the bulk of the cancer-preventing properties in apples are in the peel.

ꙮ Sliced apples freeze well in airtight containers. Frozen apples become mushy when thawed; they work well in baked goods and smoothies.

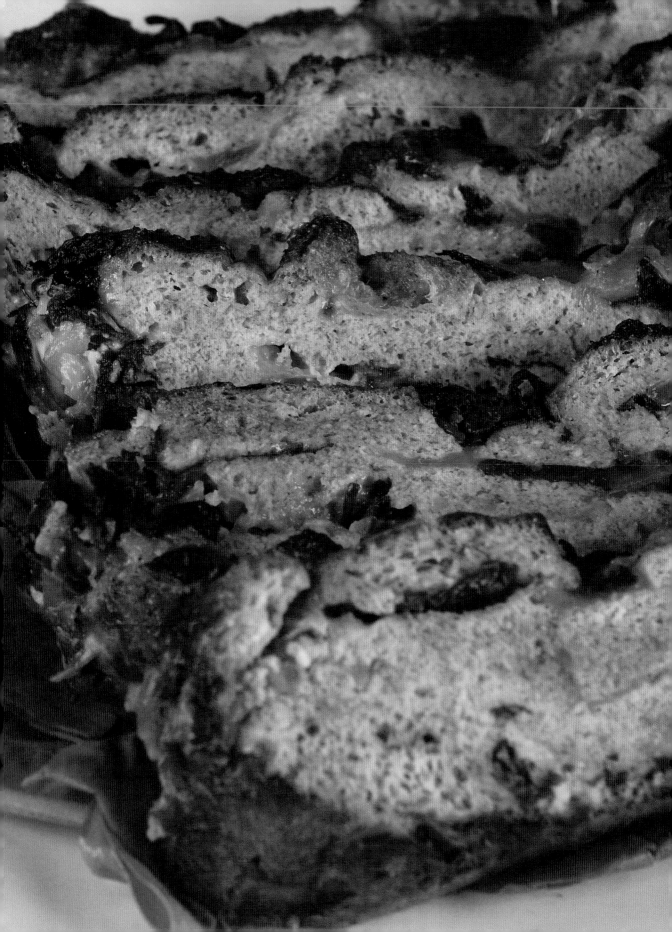

# Cheesy Spinach Squares

Estimated preparation and cooking time: 1 hour and 15 minutes

## INGREDIENTS

10 slices whole grain sandwich bread

2 teaspoons olive oil

1 large onion, diced

7 ounces fresh baby spinach, washed

6 eggs, whisked

½ cup skim milk

1 cup shredded sharp cheddar cheese

¼ teaspoon salt

¼ teaspoon black pepper

Nonstick cooking spray

ɣ Spinach is an excellent source of vitamins A, C, K and fiber; it is loaded with antioxidants!

ɣ Enjoy spinach raw and cooked. Raw spinach makes an excellent salad and can be a healthy substitute for lettuce. Steamed spinach makes a great side dish and an excellent omelet ingredient or pizza topping! We even use spinach in one of our smoothies (see page 123).

ɣ Eating spinach may help to protect us against osteoporosis, heart disease, colon cancer, and arthritis.

ɣ Cheesy Spinach Squares make a great breakfast or picnic food. They are delicious both hot and cold.

ɣ Calorie for calorie, spinach and other dark leafy greens provide more vitamins and minerals than any other foods.

## PROCEDURE

1. Preheat oven to 375°F. Lightly coat 9 x 13-inch baking dish with cooking spray.

2. Toast bread and cut or tear into ½-inch squares. Place squares in large mixing bowl.

3. In medium-sized skillet, heat olive oil on medium-high. Add diced onion and sauté until lightly brown.

4. Add spinach leaves to skillet and heat just until wilted. Add spinach and onions to toasted bread in large mixing bowl.

5. Add whisked eggs, milk, shredded cheese, salt, and pepper to mixture in large bowl. Stir until well combined.

6. Evenly spread mixture in baking dish.

7. Bake 40–45 minutes or until eggs are well cooked and bread is golden brown.

8. Allow to cool slightly. Cut into squares and enjoy.

Yield: 10 servings

## NUTRITION INFORMATION

Serving size: ¹/₁₀ recipe

Per serving: 180 calories, 8 g total fat, 3 g saturated fat, 120 mg cholesterol, 16 g carbohydrates, 4 g fiber, 4 g sugars, 12 g protein, and 280 mg sodium

CACFP: ¹/₁₀ recipe meets the snack requirement.

# Whole Wheat Pumpkin (or Squash) Muffins

Estimated preparation and cooking time: 30 minutes

## INGREDIENTS

2 eggs

½ cup sugar

1 cup canned pumpkin or puréed cooked squash

2 tablespoons canola oil

¼ cup water

2 cups white whole wheat flour

1 teaspoon baking powder

½ teaspoon baking soda

½ teaspoon salt

½ teaspoon ground cinnamon

¼ teaspoon ground nutmeg

¼ teaspoon ground cloves

½ cup raisins (optional)

Nonstick cooking spray

## PROCEDURE

1. Preheat oven to 400°F.

2. Spray muffin pan with nonstick cooking spray.

3. In large bowl, whisk eggs; add sugar, pumpkin (or squash), oil, and water; mix well.

4. In small bowl, mix flour, baking powder, soda, salt, and spices.

5. Add dry ingredients to first mixture and mix only until dry ingredients are moistened. Stir in raisins, if desired.

6. Spoon batter into muffin pan, filling each cup ⅔ full.

7. Bake 15–18 minutes.

Yield: 12 muffins

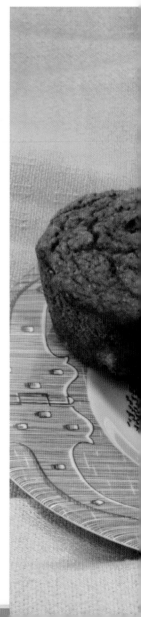

## NUTRITION INFORMATION

Serving size: 1 muffin

Per serving: 150 calories, 3½ grams total fat, 0 g saturated fat, 30 mg cholesterol, 26 g carbohydrates, 3 g fiber, 9 g sugars, 4 g protein, and 200 mg sodium

CACFP: Serve with ½ cup fluid milk, ½ cup fruit or vegetable, ½ ounce cheese, or 2 ounces yogurt.

⸙ You can make these muffins with canned, fresh, or frozen pumpkin or squash. If using fresh or frozen, you'll need to cook and purée it.

⸙ Pumpkin is rich in vitamins and minerals, including vitamins A, E, and C and potassium and iron. It is also high in fiber and contains the phytonutrient lutein, which contributes to eye health.

⸙ The largest pumpkin ever grown weighed 1,810 pounds, but the best pumpkins for cooking are the small sugar pumpkins that weigh only a few pounds.

⸙ Stirring the batter just until the dry ingredients are moistened prevents tunnels from forming in the muffins and keeps them tender. It's okay if small lumps remain in the batter.

⸙ American-style muffins have been made since the 1800s, while yeast-raised English muffins are more than 800 years old.

⸙ These muffins are also great for breakfast.

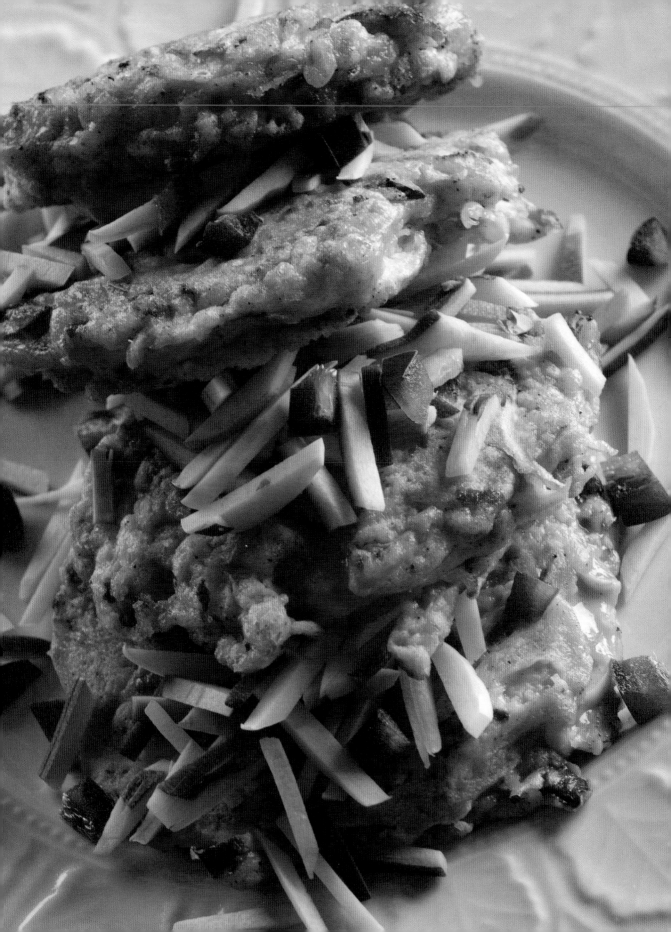

# Vegetable Fritters

Estimated preparation and cooking time: 35 minutes

## INGREDIENTS

2 large carrots

2 medium zucchini (about 10 ounces each)

2 medium summer squash (about 10 ounces each)

1 cup white whole wheat or whole wheat pastry flour

⅔ cup sharp cheddar cheese, shredded

½ teaspoon salt

½ teaspoon ground black pepper

4 large eggs, lightly beaten

Nonstick cooking spray

## PROCEDURE

1.  With coarse shredder or food processor, shred carrot, zucchini, and squash.

2.  In medium bowl, mix shredded vegetables with flour, cheese, salt, pepper, and eggs.

3.  Spray large nonstick skillet lightly with nonstick cooking spray and heat on medium or use electric griddle set at 325°F.

4.  Gently drop ¼ cup servings of vegetable mixture into skillet, flattening each fritter slightly to about 3 inches in diameter.

5.  Cook several fritters at a time, turning every 4–5 minutes, until golden brown.

6.  Serve slightly cooled or keep warm in low oven until all are cooked.

Yield: 15 servings

## NUTRITION INFORMATION

Serving size: 2 fritters; ¼ cup each

Per serving: 90 calories, 3 g total fat, 1 g saturated fat, 50 mg cholesterol, 10 g carbohydrates, 2 g fiber, 2 g sugars, 6 g protein, and 140 mg sodium

CACFP: Serve with ½ cup fluid milk or ½ slice whole grain bread.

ʄ Traditionally, fritters are sweet or savory and deep fried. Ours is a healthier version that tastes just as good.

ʄ Zucchini and summer squash are members of the same vegetable family and are rich in many nutrients, including fiber, B vitamins, vitamin C, magnesium, and potassium.

ʄ Using sharply flavored cheese allows you to use less cheese without compromising the taste of the fritters. You can also use cheese made from 1 percent or 2 percent milk as a healthier alternative to full-fat cheese.

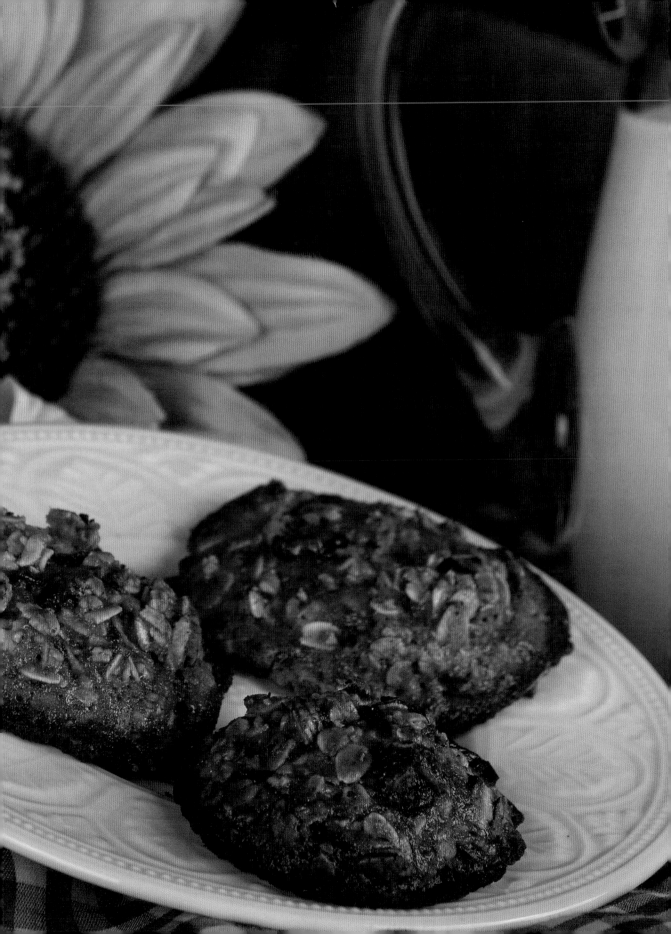

# Zucchini-Oatmeal Cookies

Estimated preparation and cooking time: 30 minutes

## INGREDIENTS

1¼ cups white whole wheat flour or whole wheat pastry flour

2 cups rolled oats

1 teaspoon baking powder

1 teaspoon ground cinnamon

¼ cup canola oil

2 tablespoons low-fat plain yogurt

1 cup brown sugar

2 large eggs

2½ teaspoons vanilla extract

1½ cups shredded zucchini

¾ cup dried cranberries (optional)

Nonstick cooking spray

## PROCEDURE

1. Preheat oven to 375°F.

2. In large bowl, combine flour, oats, baking powder, baking soda, and cinnamon. Stir until evenly combined.

3. In medium bowl, combine oil, yogurt, brown sugar, eggs, and vanilla. Whisk until well combined. Then gently fold in shredded zucchini.

4. Create well in middle of dry ingredients and slowly add wet ingredients. Stir until evenly combined. If using, gently fold in dried cranberries.

5. Lightly coat cookie sheets with cooking spray.

6. Drop dough onto cookie sheets, using teaspoon. Space cookies about 2 inches apart, making 20 cookies.

7. Bake 10–12 minutes or until golden brown.

8. Allow to cool and enjoy!

Yield: 20 cookies

## NUTRITION INFORMATION

Serving size: 1 cookie

Per serving: 150 calories, 4 g total fat, 0 g saturated fat, 20 mg cholesterol, 27 g carbohydrates, 2 g fiber, 14 g sugars, 3 g protein, and 30 mg sodium

CACFP: Serve with ½ cup fluid milk, ½ cup fruit, or 2 ounces yogurt.

⸕ Mild-tasting zucchini is a very versatile vegetable. You can use it in soups, salads, casseroles, breads, cakes, and cookies.

⸕ Whole grain flour and oats, canola oil, and zucchini make these cookies a healthy variation of a favorite snack.

⸕ The word *cookie* comes from an old Dutch word meaning "little cake."

# Cinnamon & Vanilla Yogurt Dip

Estimated preparation time: 5 minutes

## INGREDIENTS

1 cup low-fat vanilla yogurt (or vanilla soy yogurt)

½ teaspoon ground cinnamon

## PROCEDURE

**Stir together until well mixed.**

Yield: 10 servings

These dips add nutrition and fun to snacktime. Serve one or more of the dips with 5 cups of assorted fresh fruit, such as pears, apples, strawberries, bananas, peaches, nectarines, melon, oranges, or pineapple.

## NUTRITION INFORMATION

Serving size: ⅒ recipe

Per serving (dip only): 20 calories, 0 g total fat, 0 g saturated fat, 0 mg cholesterol, 3 g carbohydrates, 0 g fiber, 3 g sugars, 1 g protein, and 15 mg sodium

CACFP: Serve fresh fruit with ½ ounce nuts (if allowed at your center) per child, whole grain crackers or pretzels, or 1 Early Sprouts muffin to create a complete snack. Or provide each child with ½ cup fluid milk.

Select fruits of various colors. Different-colored fruits (and vegetables) offer different vitamins, minerals, and phytonutrients (cancer-fighting properties).

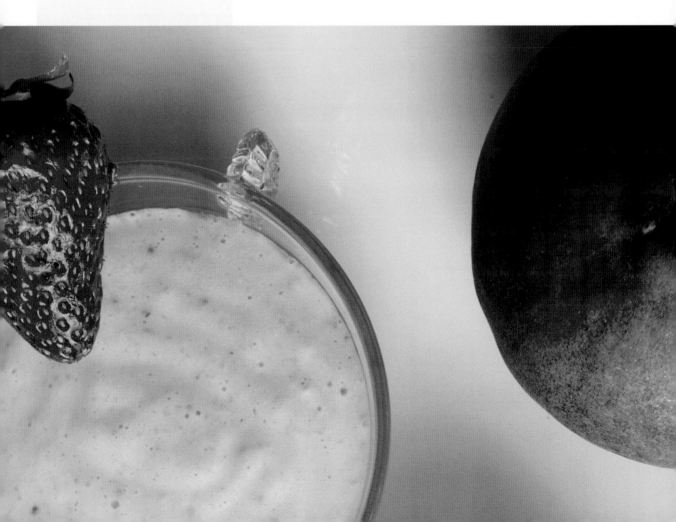

# Strawberry Yogurt Dip

Estimated preparation time: 5 minutes

## INGREDIENTS

2 cups fresh strawberries (or thawed frozen strawberries)

1 cup low-fat vanilla yogurt

¼ cup reduced-fat cream cheese

↳ Select in-season fruit. When fruits are in season, they are less expensive and at their freshest.

## PROCEDURE

**Combine all ingredients in food processor or blender; mix until smooth.**

Yield: 10 servings

## NUTRITION INFORMATION

Serving size: ¹⁄₁₀ recipe

Per serving (dip only): 45 calories, 1½ g total fat, 1 g saturated fat, 5 mg cholesterol, 6 g carbohydrates, <1 g fiber, 5 g sugars, 2 g protein, and 35 mg sodium

CACFP: Serve the fresh fruit with ½ ounce nuts (if allowed at your center) per child, whole grain crackers or pretzels, or 1 Early Sprouts muffin to create a complete snack. Or provide each child with ½ cup fluid milk.

# Strawberry Soy Yogurt Dip

Estimated preparation time: 5 minutes      (DAIRY FREE)

## INGREDIENTS

2 cups fresh strawberries (or thawed frozen strawberries)

1 cup vanilla soy yogurt

↳ Squeeze a fresh lemon, lime, or orange juice onto sliced apples, pears, and other fruits prone to browning to help maintain the fruit's natural color.

## PROCEDURE

**Combine all ingredients in food processor or blender; mix until smooth.**

Yield: 10 servings

## NUTRITION INFORMATION

Serving size: ¹⁄₁₀ recipe

Per serving (dip only): 25 calories, 0 g total fat, 0 g saturated fat, 0 mg cholesterol, 4 g carbohydrates, <1 g fiber, 3 g sugars, 1 g protein, and 0 mg sodium

CACFP: Serve the fresh fruit with ½ ounce nuts (if allowed at your center) per child, whole grain crackers or pretzels, or 1 Early Sprouts muffin to create a complete snack. Or provide each child with ½ cup fluid milk.

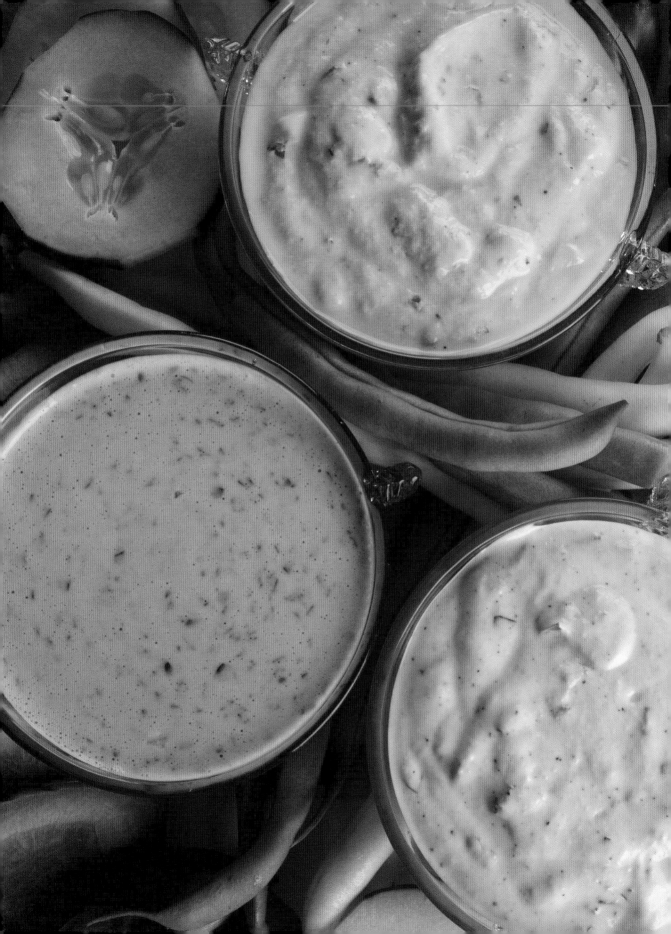

# Veggie Herb Dip

Estimated preparation time: 5 minutes

## INGREDIENTS

1½ cups plain low- or nonfat yogurt, Greek yogurt, or yogurt cheese

½ cup low-fat mayonnaise

½ teaspoon salt

2 teaspoons each dried dill, parsley, and chives (use fresh if available)

2 teaspoons fresh lemon juice

½ teaspoon garlic powder

½ teaspoon paprika

These veggie dips add fun and flavor to nutritious snacks. Serve one or more of the veggie dips with 5 cups of sliced bell peppers, broccoli, cauliflower, carrots, cucumbers, cherry tomatoes, zucchini, summer squash, or green beans. Wash and slice the vegetables as needed. Serve dip in individual small bowls.

## PROCEDURE

**Combine ingredients in small mixing bowl; stir until evenly combined. Chill 1 hour and serve with vegetables.**

Yield: 10 servings

## NUTRITION INFORMATION

Serving size: $1/10$ recipe

Per serving (dip only): 40 calories, 2½ g total fat, 0 g saturated fat, 5 mg cholesterol, 3 g carbohydrates, 0 g fiber, 2 g sugars, 1 g protein, and 100 mg sodium

CACFP: Serve with ½ ounce whole grain crackers.

⚬ **If you prefer a thicker dip, replace the yogurt with yogurt cheese. To make yogurt cheese, tie yogurt securely in cheesecloth over a bowl or line a strainer with cheesecloth or a coffee filter and drain yogurt for 1–2 hours or overnight in the refrigerator. Scrape the thickened yogurt (yogurt cheese) from the cheesecloth and enjoy! Yogurt cheese can also be a healthy substitute for cream cheese in many recipes.**

# Spinach Dip

Estimated preparation time: 5 minutes

## INGREDIENTS

1 cup baby spinach leaves

½ cup low-fat plain yogurt

½ cup cooked or canned chickpeas

⅛ teaspoon garlic powder

⅛ sweet onion (such as Vidalia), chopped

⅛ teaspoon salt

⚬ **Dips made with dairy products or other perishable ingredients should be served as soon as they are prepared. Otherwise store them in the refrigerator for later use.**

## PROCEDURE

**Combine ingredients in food processor or powerful blender. Mix until combined.**

Yield: 10 servings

## NUTRITION INFORMATION

Serving size: $1/10$ recipe

Per serving (dip only): 25 calories, 0 g total fat, 0 g saturated fat, 0 mg cholesterol, 4 g carbohydrates, <1 g fiber, 1 g sugar, 1 g protein, and 40 mg sodium

CACFP: Serve with ½ ounce whole grain crackers.

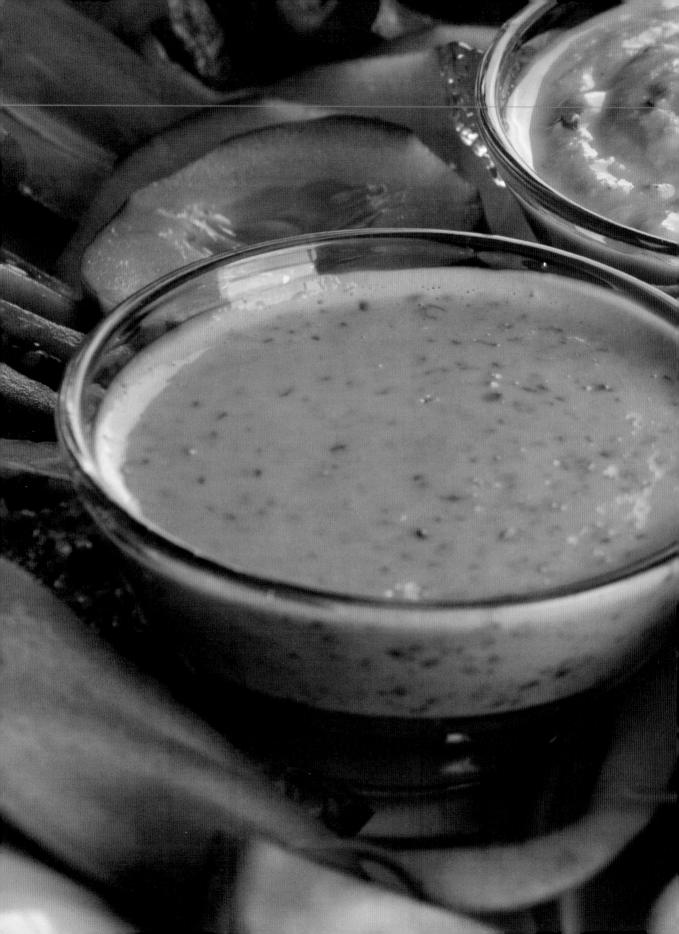

# Yogurt Ranch Dip

Estimated preparation time: 5 minutes

## INGREDIENTS

1 cup low-fat plain yogurt

½ cup low-fat mayonnaise

¼ teaspoon dried parsley

⅛ teaspoon garlic powder

⅛ teaspoon sea salt

¼ teaspoon black pepper

2 tablespoons fresh chives, finely chopped

## PROCEDURE

**Place ingredients in medium mixing bowl; stir vigorously until evenly combined. Chill first or serve with vegetables.**

## NUTRITION INFORMATION

Serving size: ¹⁄₁₀ recipe

Per serving (dip only): 50 calories, 3½ g total fat, ½ g saturated fat, 5 mg cholesterol, 3 g carbohydrates, 0 g fiber, 2 g sugars, 1 g protein, and 115 mg sodium

CACFP: Serve with ½ ounce whole grain crackers.

**⸕ You can encourage experimentation by serving two or more different vegetables to dip, and children can compare how the dip tastes with them. You can also serve two or more different dips with a single vegetable and have the children decide which dip they prefer with that vegetable.**

# Soy Ranch Dip

Estimated preparation time: 5 minutes    (DAIRY FREE)

## INGREDIENTS

12-ounce package silken tofu

2 teaspoons fresh lemon juice

¼ teaspoon salt

⅛ teaspoon black pepper

1 teaspoon dried parsley

1 teaspoon onion powder

¼ teaspoon garlic powder

**⸕ Finding a dip that children like is often a great way to increase their vegetable consumption. Unfortunately, most dips are high in fat and cholesterol. We hope you will find a favorite among our healthy dip recipes.**

## PROCEDURE

**Place ingredients in blender or food processor; mix until smooth and well combined. Chill first or serve with vegetables.**

Yield: 10 servings

## NUTRITION INFORMATION

Serving size: ¹⁄₁₀ recipe

Per serving (dip only): 25 calories, 1 g total fat, 0 g saturated fat, 0 mg cholesterol, 1 g carbohydrates, 0 g fiber, 0 g sugar, 2 g protein, and 75 mg sodium

CACFP: Serve with ½ ounce whole grain crackers.

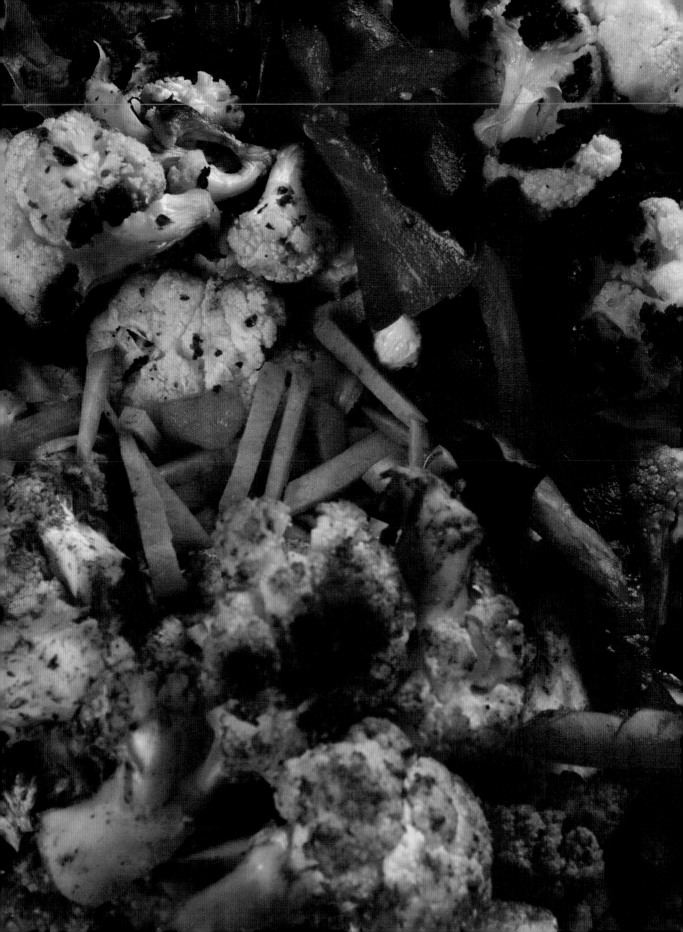

# Italian-Style Roasted Cauliflower

Estimated preparation and cooking time: 50 minutes

## INGREDIENTS

1 large head cauliflower (yields about 8 cups raw florets)

2 tablespoons canola oil

1 teaspoon dried basil

1 teaspoon dried marjoram

1 teaspoon dried oregano

¼ teaspoon garlic powder

½ teaspoon salt

Nonstick cooking spray

## PROCEDURE

1. Preheat oven to 400°F. Coat large, rimmed baking pan with nonstick cooking spray.

2. Cut cauliflower into quarters and remove core. Cut cauliflower into bite-sized florets.

3. In large bowl, combine canola oil with basil, marjoram, oregano, garlic powder, and salt.

4. Add cauliflower florets and toss gently to coat evenly with oil and spice mixture.

5. Spread cauliflower evenly in prepared baking pan. Bake 30–40 minutes, stirring after 15–20 minutes. Cauliflower should be tender and golden brown. Allow to cool slightly and serve.

Yield: 16 servings

## NUTRITION INFORMATION

Serving size: ½ cup

Per serving: 25 calories, 2 g total fat, 0 g saturated fat, 0 mg cholesterol, 2 g carbohydrates, 1 g fiber, 1 g sugars, 1 g protein, and 80 mg sodium

CACFP: Serve with ½ cup fluid milk, ⅓ cup dry cereal, ½ ounce cheese, or 2 ounces yogurt.

⊬ Despite its white color, cauliflower is a very good source of vitamin C, vitamin B6, folate, and fiber.

⊬ Cauliflower is a cruciferous vegetable—the crucifers are a family of vegetables that includes broccoli, cabbage, and kale. Cruciferous vegetables contain compounds that may help prevent cancer.

⊬ The head (or curd) of a cauliflower is made up of undeveloped flower buds.

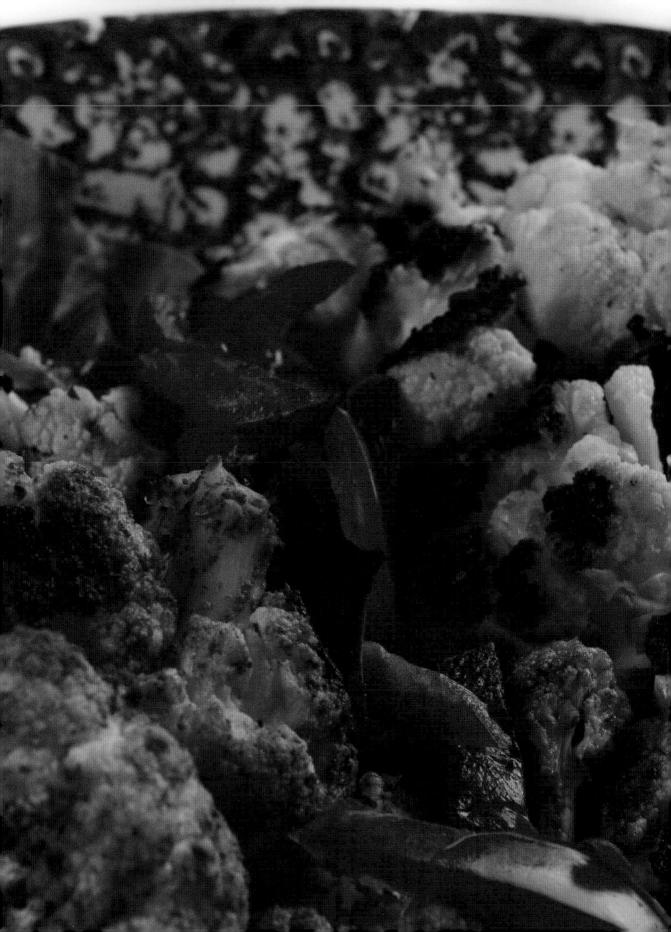

# Indian-Style Roasted Cauliflower

Estimated preparation and cooking time: 50 minutes

## INGREDIENTS

1 large head cauliflower (yields about 8 cups raw florets)

¼ teaspoon ground coriander

½ teaspoon ground cumin

¼ teaspoon turmeric

¼ teaspoon ground cardamom

¼ teaspoon ground cinnamon

¼ teaspoon ground cloves

½ teaspoon salt

2 tablespoons canola oil

Nonstick cooking spray

## PROCEDURE

1. Preheat oven to 400°F. Coat large, rimmed baking pan with nonstick cooking spray.

2. Cut cauliflower into quarters and remove core. Cut cauliflower into bite-sized florets.

3. In large bowl, combine the spice mixture—ground coriander, cumin, turmeric, cardamom, cinnamon, cloves, and salt—with canola oil. Stir well.

4. Add cauliflower florets and toss gently until florets are evenly coated with oil and spice mixture.

5. Spread cauliflower evenly in prepared baking pan. Bake 30–40 minutes, stirring after 15–20 minutes. Cauliflower should be tender and golden brown. Allow to cool slightly and serve.

Yield: 16 servings

## NUTRITION INFORMATION

Serving size: ½ cup

Per serving: 25 calories, 2 g total fat, 0 g saturated fat, 0 mg cholesterol, 2 g carbohydrates, 1 g fiber, 1 g sugars, 1 g protein, and 80 mg sodium

CACFP: Serve with ½ cup fluid milk, ⅓ cup dry cereal, ½ ounce cheese, or 2 ounces yogurt.

⋮ Cauliflower isn't just white anymore—you can now find orange, green, and even purple heads. Enjoying these cauliflowers is a nice way to add color and nutrition to your plate.

⋮ Orange cauliflower boasts much higher levels of vitamin A, which helps promote healthy skin.

⋮ Green cauliflower is also called *broccoflower*.

⋮ Purple cauliflower gets its color from the same heart-healthy antioxidant found in blueberries, red cabbage, and eggplant.

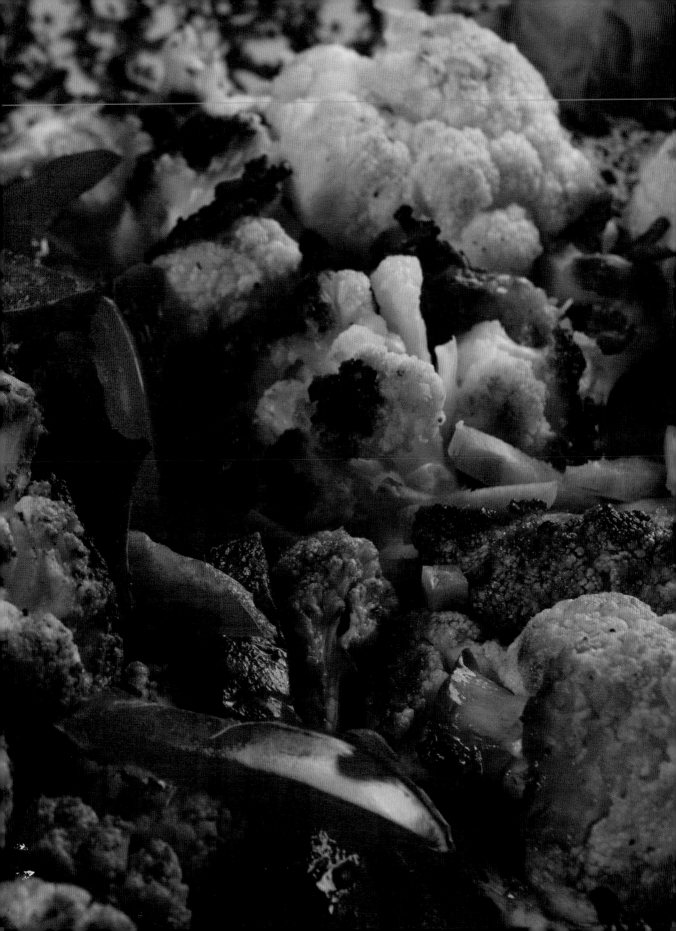

# Dijon-Parmesan Roasted Cauliflower

Estimated preparation and cooking time: 50 minutes

## INGREDIENTS

1 large head cauliflower (yields about 8 cups raw florets)

1 tablespoon Dijon mustard

½ teaspoon salt

2 tablespoons Parmesan cheese

¼ teaspoon garlic powder

2 tablespoons canola oil

Nonstick cooking spray

## PROCEDURE

1. Preheat oven to 400°F. Coat large, rimmed baking pan with nonstick cooking spray.

2. Cut cauliflower into quarters and remove core. Cut cauliflower into bite-sized florets.

3. In large bowl, combine mustard, salt, Parmesan, and garlic powder with canola oil; mix well.

4. Add cauliflower florets and toss gently until florets are evenly coated with mixture.

5. Spread cauliflower evenly in prepared baking pan. Bake 30–40 minutes, stirring after 15–20 minutes. Cauliflower should be tender and golden brown. Allow to cool slightly and serve.

Yield: 16 servings

## NUTRITION INFORMATION

Serving size: ½ cup

Per serving: 30 calories, 2 g total fat, 0 g saturated fat, 0 mg cholesterol, 2 g carbohydrates, 1 g fiber, 1 g sugars, 1 g protein, and 105 mg sodium

CACFP: Serve with ½ cup fluid milk, ⅓ cup dry cereal, ½ ounce cheese, or 2 ounces yogurt.

⸎ In 1856 Jean Naigeon of Dijon, France, made the first version of what is now called Dijon mustard. Instead of adding vinegar to the traditional mustard recipe, Naigeon used verjuice, which is juice from grapes that aren't quite ripe.

⸎ Cauliflower takes its name from the Latin word for cabbage, *caulis*, and the word *flower*.

⸎ California produces about 90 percent of all the cauliflower grown in the United States.

⸎ The United States has about 35,000 acres of land used to grow cauliflower.

# Honey-Balsamic Roasted Cauliflower

Estimated preparation and cooking time: 50 minutes

## INGREDIENTS

1 large head cauliflower (yields about 8 cups raw florets)

1 tablespoon canola oil

1 tablespoon honey

2 tablespoons balsamic vinegar

½ teaspoon salt

Nonstick cooking spray

## PROCEDURE

1. Preheat oven to 400°F. Coat large, rimmed baking pan with nonstick cooking spray.

2. Cut cauliflower into quarters and remove core. Cut cauliflower into bite-sized florets.

3. Place oil and honey in large, microwavable bowl. Warm in microwave 10 seconds. Mix in balsamic vinegar and salt.

4. Add cauliflower florets and toss gently until florets are evenly coated with honey, vinegar, and oil mixture.

5. Spread cauliflower evenly in prepared baking pan. Bake 30–40 minutes, stirring after 15–20 minutes. Cauliflower should be tender and golden brown. Allow to cool slightly and serve.

Yield: 16 servings

## NUTRITION INFORMATION

Serving size: ½ cup

Per serving: 25 calories, 1 g total fat, 0 g saturated fat, 0 mg cholesterol, 3 g carbohydrates, 1 g fiber, 2 g sugars, 1 g protein, and 80 mg sodium

CACFP: Serve with ½ cup fluid milk, ⅓ cup dry cereal, ½ ounce cheese, or 2 ounces yogurt.

- Enjoy cauliflower raw, steamed, boiled, or roasted.

- Cauliflower is believed to have its origins in Asia Minor.

- Cauliflower has been eaten in the Mediterranean region since 600 BCE.

- Pickled cauliflower is often included in Italian antipasto platters.

- The humorist and author Mark Twain wrote, "Cauliflower is nothing but cabbage with a college education."

# Roasted Root Vegetables

Estimated preparation and cooking time: 50 minutes

## INGREDIENTS

5 cups carrots and parsnips

2 teaspoons canola oil

¼ teaspoon salt

Pepper to taste

⊦ Other root vegetables, such as beets and sweet potatoes, can also be used.

⊦ Look for small, firm, and well-shaped root vegetables. Root vegetables that are too large tend to have a woody texture and are not as sweet.

⊦ Carrots are grown around the world in a variety of colors, including purple, white, and yellow!

⊦ If you purchase carrots that still have their green tops, be sure to remove the tops before storing. The tops will cause the carrots to wilt because they pull moisture from the roots.

⊦ Raw parsnips, despite their white color, are an excellent source of vitamin C. Parsnips are also high in folate and a good source of potassium.

⊦ The first frost of the season converts some of the starch in parsnips to sugar, giving them a sweeter taste.

## PROCEDURE

1. Preheat oven to 425°F. Lightly coat baking sheet with oil.

2. Scrub all root vegetables well, using vegetable brush. Trim tops.

3. Steam whole carrots and parsnips until just tender.

4. Cut vegetables into long, thin strips and place in large bowl.

5. Gently coat vegetables with canola or other vegetable oil.

6. Spread evenly in baking dish. Season with salt and pepper.

7. Bake 30–45 minutes (flipping every 10–15 minutes) until golden brown.

Yield: 10 servings

## NUTRITION INFORMATION

Serving size: ½ cup vegetables

Per serving: 50 calories, 1½ g total fat, 0 g saturated fat, 0 mg cholesterol, 9 g carbohydrates, 2 g fiber, 3 g sugars, 1 g protein, and 70 mg sodium

CACFP: Serve with ½ ounce whole grain crackers.

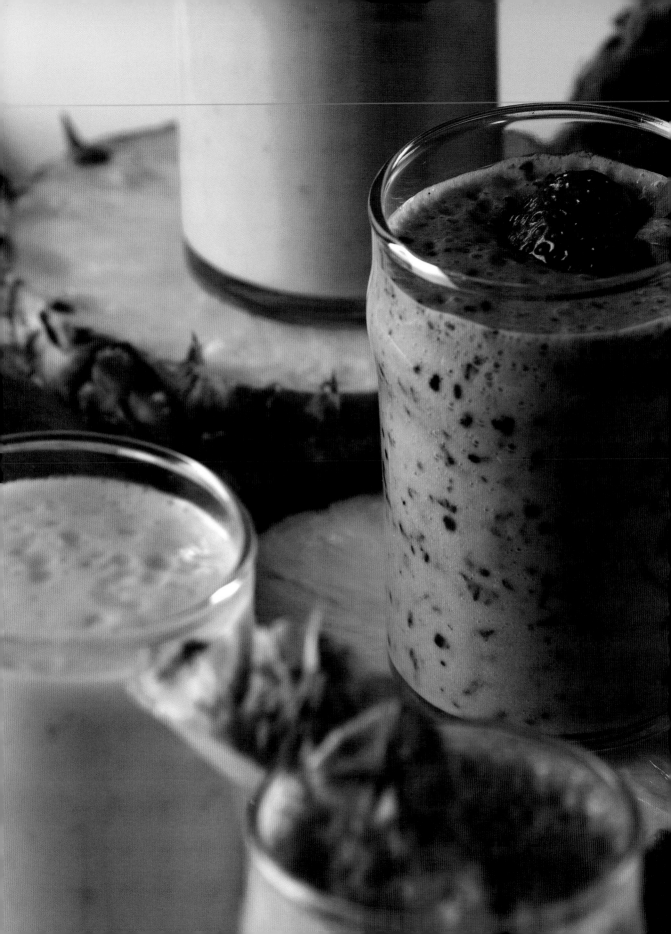

# Berry-Banana Smoothie

Estimated preparation time: 5 minutes

## INGREDIENTS

3 cups skim milk

1½ cups low-fat vanilla yogurt

1½ cups thawed frozen or fresh blueberries (blackberries, strawberries, or raspberries also work great)

1 large banana

⸋ **Experiment with different types of fruits and vegetables in your smoothie. Always include a banana, because it does wonders for the texture.**

## PROCEDURE

**Blend all ingredients until well combined. Depending on size of blender, you may need to make this in two batches.**

Yield: 10 servings

## NUTRITION INFORMATION

Serving size: ¹/₁₀ recipe

Per serving: 70 calories, ½ g total fat, 0 g saturated fat, 5 mg cholesterol, 12 g carbohydrates, <1 g fiber, 11 g sugars, 5 g protein, and 55 mg sodium

CACFP: Serve with ½ ounce whole grain crackers or pretzels.

Smoothies are like a meal in a cup, offering carbohydrates, protein, and a small amount of fat. Here are some smoothie recipes that are sure to please.

# Mango Smoothie

Estimated preparation time: 5 minutes

## INGREDIENTS

3 cups skim milk

1½ cups low-fat vanilla yogurt

1½ cups thawed frozen or fresh mango (peach also works great)

1 large banana

⸋ **Smoothies are a rich source of bone-building calcium. They are also a great way to encourage children to eat more fruits and vegetables.**

## PROCEDURE

**Blend all ingredients until well combined. Depending on size of blender, you may need to make this in two batches.**

Yield: 10 servings

## NUTRITION INFORMATION

Serving size: ¹/₁₀ recipe

Per serving: 70 calories, ½ g total fat, 0 g saturated fat, 5 mg cholesterol, 13 g carbohydrate, <1 g fiber, 13 g sugars, 5 g protein, and 55 mg sodium

CACFP: Serve with ½ ounce whole grain crackers or pretzels.

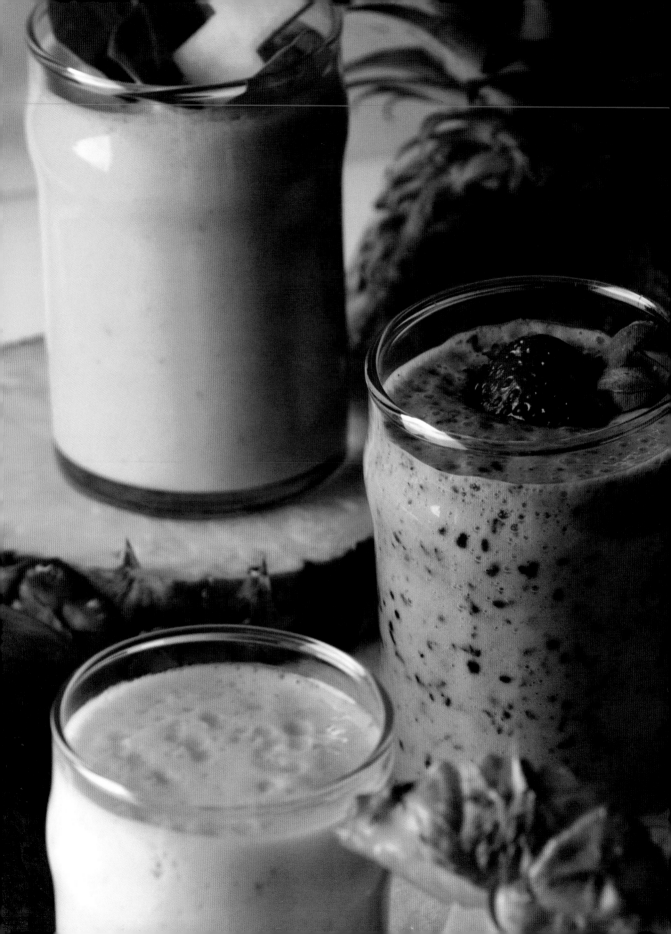

# Banana–Butternut Squash Smoothie

Estimated preparation time: 5 minutes

## INGREDIENTS

3 cups skim milk

1½ cups low-fat vanilla yogurt

1½ cups cooked butternut squash
   (make sure it has cooled first)

1 large banana

1½ teaspoon vanilla extract

1 teaspoon ground cinnamon

☞ **Add nut butters, tofu, wheat germ, or ground flax seed for a nutritional boost!**

## PROCEDURE

**Blend all ingredients until well combined. Depending on size of blender, you may need to make this in two batches.**

Yield: 10 servings

## NUTRITION INFORMATION

Serving size: ¹/₁₀ recipe

Per serving: 70 calories, ½ g total fat, 0 g saturated fat, 5 mg cholesterol, 13 g carbohydrates, 1 g fiber, 9 g sugars, 5 g protein, and 55 mg sodium

CACFP: Serve with ½ ounce whole grain crackers or pretzels.

# Pineapple-Spinach Smoothie

Estimated preparation time: 5 minutes

*This is a good beverage to serve to your experienced smoothie drinkers.*

## INGREDIENTS

3 cups skim milk

1½ cup low-fat plain yogurt

1 cup crushed pineapple (fresh or canned in water)

2 cups fresh baby spinach leaves

1 large banana

☞ **Smoothies became famous during the 1960s, along with juice bars, tofu, and granola!**

## PROCEDURE

**Blend all ingredients until well combined. Depending on size of blender, you may need to make this in two batches.**

Yield: 10 servings

## NUTRITION INFORMATION

Serving size: ¹/₁₀ recipe

Per serving: 60 calories, ½ g total fat, 0 g saturated fat, 5 mg cholesterol, 9 g carbohydrates, <1 g fiber, 8 g sugars, 5 g protein, and 65 mg sodium

CACFP: Serve with ½ ounce whole grain crackers or pretzels.

# EIGHT

# RECIPES
## FOR
# CELEBRATIONS

WHEN WE THINK ABOUT CELEBRATIONS, one of the first things that comes to mind is food. Our culture strongly associates celebrations with treat foods—cookies at Christmas, candy at Halloween, and cake and ice cream for birthdays. For preschool staff, trying to achieve a balance between a family's desire to celebrate special occasions with traditional treats and the wish to do what's best for children can be challenging.

As more preschools make a commitment to serving healthier foods, many are establishing nutrition policies that exclude foods brought from home. This can be difficult for parents, for they may want to celebrate with their children as they wish. Similarly, many parents feel they should have some control over what foods their children are offered. Finding out that the morning snack consisted of frosted cupcakes may be upsetting to a parent who is trying to keep her child's diet as healthy as possible.

Starting to separate food from celebration is an effective way to deal with this mind-set. This is often easier for the children to accept than the parents! Children love a party, and celebrating with activities and nonfood items can be as exciting as cake and ice cream. Encourage parents to send in nonfood items, such as stickers or inexpensive toys. Better yet, invite parents to visit the classroom on the special day for a game or a fun activity. Having parents visit school is a huge treat for children.

Another approach is to help children (and parents) start associating celebrations with healthier foods. This chapter includes seasonal foods that can be incorporated into the holidays you observe. For birthday parties, fruit or veggie platters with dip, a child's favorite healthy food, or healthier versions of traditional party foods can be effective. The two cake recipes presented here are popular selections from the Early Sprouts curriculum that have been adapted for baking as birthday cakes. Both are made with whole wheat flour, healthy oils, and vegetables. No frosting is necessary. Children love them just as they are.

# Gingerbread Pancakes

Estimated preparation and cooking time: 25 minutes

## INGREDIENTS

1 egg

1¼ cups skim milk

3 tablespoons molasses

2 tablespoons canola oil

1⅓ cups white whole wheat flour

1 teaspoon baking powder

¼ teaspoon baking soda

⅛ teaspoon salt

1 teaspoon ground cinnamon

½ teaspoon ground ginger

Pinch of ground cloves

Nonstick cooking spray

## PROCEDURE

1. In medium bowl, beat egg with whisk. Blend in milk, molasses, and canola oil.

2. Combine flour, baking powder, baking soda, salt, and spices in second medium bowl.

3. Add dry ingredients to wet ingredients and mix only until smooth.

4. Lightly spray nonstick skillet or electric griddle with nonstick cooking spray. Heat skillet on medium-high or electric griddle at 375°F.

5. Pour ⅛ cupful (2 tablespoons) servings onto griddle. Cook until pancakes are puffed and browned on one side; flip and cook until browned on other side.

6. Serve with Pear Applesauce (page 129).

Yield: 10 servings (20 pancakes)

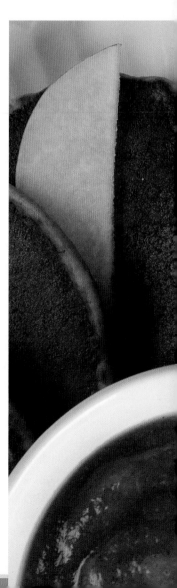

## NUTRITION INFORMATION

Serving size: 2 pancakes

Per serving: 130 calories, 3½ g total fat, 0 g saturated fat, 20 mg cholesterol, 19 g carbohydrates, 2 g fiber, 5 g sugars, 4 g protein, and 125 mg sodium

CACFP: Serve 2 Gingerbread Pancakes with ½ cup Pear Applesauce and ¾ cup fluid milk for breakfast.

- These pancakes are a healthy way to enjoy the flavors of gingerbread. They have more fiber and less sugar and fat than traditional gingerbread cake or cookies. Making them with whole wheat flour provides an additional nutrition boost.

- Gingerbread has been eaten in the United States since colonial times. According to legend, George Washington's mother served it to General Lafayette (she put orange peel in hers).

- William Shakespeare mentions gingerbread in his play *Love's Labor's Lost*: "And I had but one penny in the world, thou shouldst have it to buy ginger-bread."

- The tradition of making shapes out of gingerbread goes back to the Middle Ages. Young women believed that eating a gingerbread husband would help them find a man to marry.

- Have you ever noticed that fresh gingerroot looks like antlers? The word *ginger* comes from the Sanskrit word for "hornlike."

- Ginger has been used as a spice in many parts of the world for more than 2,000 years.

- Ginger is also valuable as a natural remedy, especially for gastrointestinal complaints. Studies have found that it may prevent motion sickness and morning sickness.

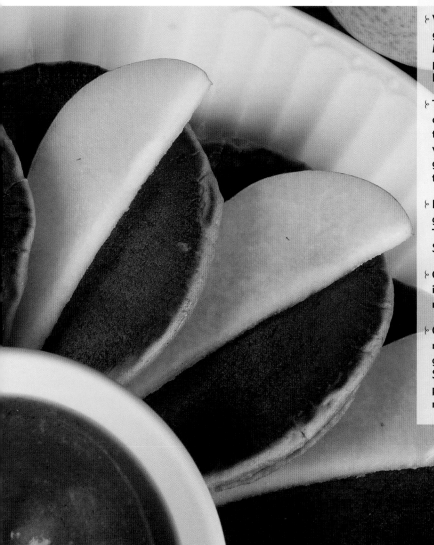

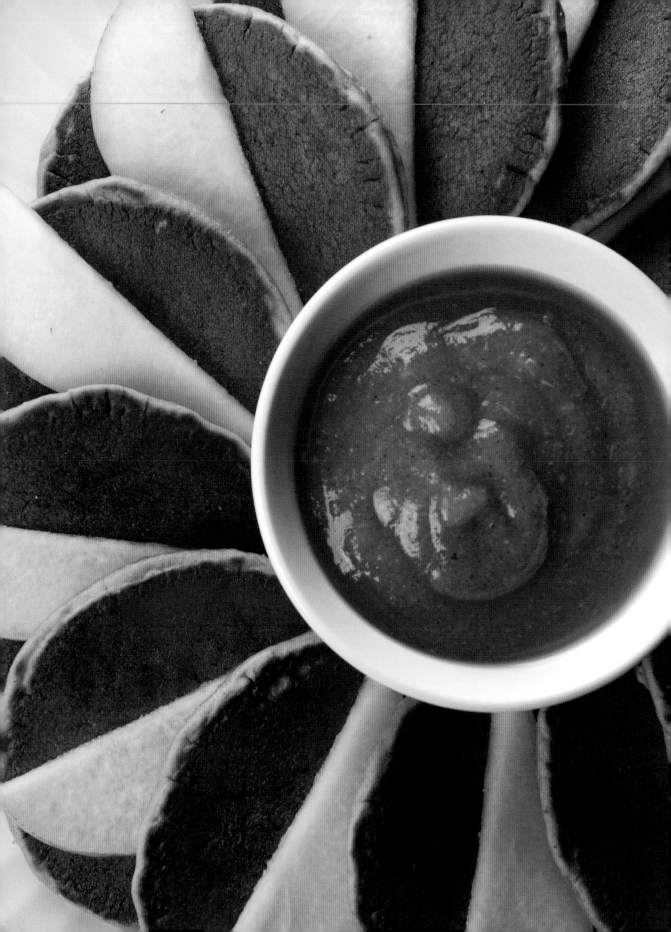

# Pear Applesauce

Estimated preparation and cooking time: 55 minutes

## INGREDIENTS

2 pounds apples

2 pounds pears

¾ cup water

1 3-inch cinnamon stick

2 teaspoons grated organic orange rind

¼ teaspoon ground cloves

¼ teaspoon ground allspice

2 teaspoons brown sugar (optional)

## PROCEDURE

1. Wash apples and pears. Cut each into 8 pieces and place in large pot. If you don't have a food mill, peel and core the fruit before cooking it, and mash it well with a potato masher after it's cooked. Add the water and cinnamon stick.

2. Bring to boil on medium-high; reduce to medium-low and cook, stirring occasionally, 30–40 minutes or until fruit is very soft.

3. Remove cinnamon stick. Use food mill to process cooked fruit into sauce.

4. Add orange rind, cloves, allspice, and brown sugar to warm sauce; mix well.

5. Cool slightly, serve, or refrigerate.

Yield: 10 servings

⋆ Warm pear applesauce is a tasty and healthy topping for pancakes, French toast, and waffles. It's also good topped with granola (page 61).

⋆ Using more than one variety of apples will make this sauce even tastier.

⋆ When serving fresh pears, wash them well and leave the skin on—it contains a large portion of the fruit's nutrients, fiber, and antioxidants.

⋆ Pears are considered hypoallergenic —that's why they're commonly one of the first foods to be introduced to babies.

⋆ Pears, like apples, are distantly related to roses.

⋆ Applesauce was the first food eaten in space by astronaut John Glenn in 1962.

## NUTRITION INFORMATION

Serving size: ½ cup

Per serving: 100 calories, ½ g total fat, 0 g saturated fat, 0 mg cholesterol, 25 g carbohydrates, 4 g fiber, 18 g sugars, 1 g protein, and 0 mg sodium

CACFP: Pear Applesauce meets the fruit/vegetable requirement for breakfast or snack with ½ cup; ¼ cup meets half of the fruit/vegetable requirement for lunch.

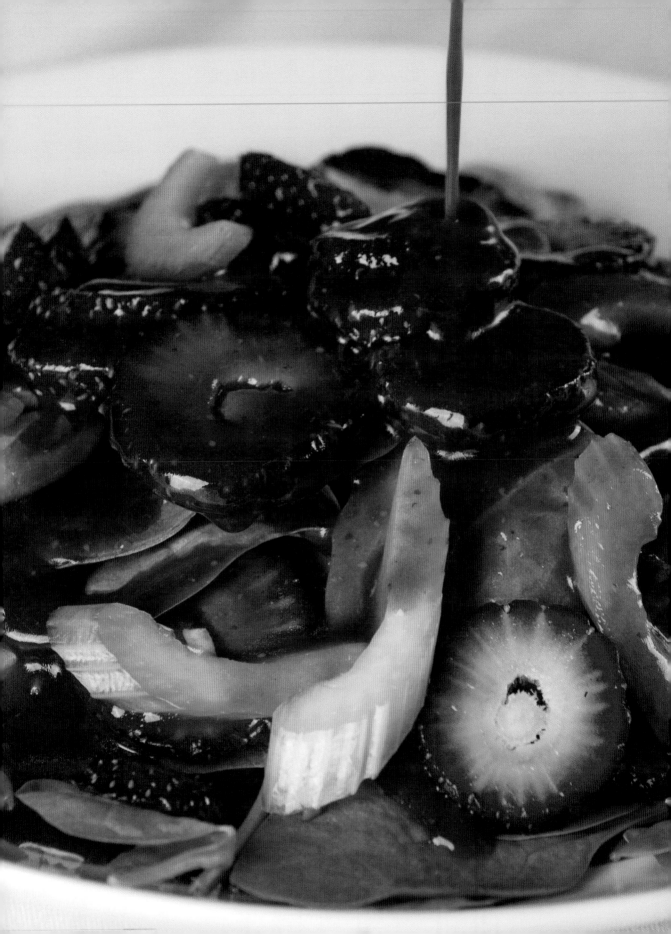

# Spinach & Strawberry Salad

Estimated preparation and cooking time: 20 minutes

## INGREDIENTS

6 tablespoons olive oil

3 tablespoons balsamic vinegar

2 tablespoons honey

1 tablespoon Dijon mustard

5 cups fresh organic baby spinach, washed

1½ cups fresh strawberries, washed and chopped

1¼ cups celery, washed and chopped

## PROCEDURE

1. Combine olive oil, balsamic vinegar, honey, and Dijon mustard in small jar with tight-fitting lid. Close lid securely and shake jar to mix ingredients.

2. Place ½ cup spinach each in 10 small bowls. Top with 2 tablespoons each strawberries and celery and 1 tablespoon dressing.

Yield: 10 servings

## NUTRITION INFORMATION

Serving size: ½ cup spinach, 2 tablespoons strawberries, 2 tablespoons celery, 1 tablespoon dressing

Per serving: 100 calories, 8 g total fat, 1 g saturated fat, 0 mg cholesterol, 8 g carbohydrates, 1 g fiber, 5 g sugars, 1 g protein, and 45 mg sodium

CACFP: Serve with ¾ cup fluid milk, ½ slice whole wheat bread, and 1½ ounces meat or meat alternate.

⹋ Fresh baby greens, such as spinach, are the first vegetables to be harvested in the spring. A salad topped with fresh berries is a nutritious way to celebrate the new season.

⹋ We recommend using organic spinach to avoid exposure to pesticides—nonorganic spinach is likely to contain high levels of pesticides that can't be washed off.

⹋ Most children love strawberries—you may want to buy extra!

⹋ Strawberries are both delicious and nutritious. They are high in fiber, vitamin C, and antioxidants.

⹋ Strawberries are very perishable and last only a day or two in the refrigerator. To avoid mold, they shouldn't be washed until you're ready to use them.

⹋ The common practice of spreading straw around the plants, which keeps the ripening berries from touching the damp ground, led to the name strawberries.

⹋ Strawberries are related to roses.

⹋ Authentic balsamic vinegar is aged in wooden barrels for at least twelve years. The balsamic vinegars that you'll find in a grocery store are produced much more quickly but still add a unique and delicious flavor to many foods.

⹋ Condiment mustard is made from the seeds of the mustard plant, which has been used for thousands of years as medicine for a variety of ailments.

# Streusel-Topped Rhubarb Coffee Cake

Estimated preparation and cooking time: 1 hour

## INGREDIENTS

### STREUSEL TOPPING

1½ tablespoons unsalted butter

¼ cup white whole wheat flour

2 tablespoons brown sugar

½ cup chopped pecans

¾ teaspoon cinnamon

### COFFEE CAKE

2 tablespoons unsalted butter

6 tablespoons plain non-fat yogurt

¾ cup sugar

1 egg

½ cup non-fat milk

1 teaspoon vanilla

1½ cups white whole wheat flour

2½ teaspoons baking powder

1½ teaspoons cinnamon

2 cups of ¼-inch pieces of rhubarb

Nonstick cooking spray

## PROCEDURE

1. Preheat oven to 350°F. Using nonstick spray, grease a 10-inch round cake pan.

2. In a small bowl, mix all streusel topping ingredients together with a fork until crumbly. Set aside.

3. In a second small mixing bowl, cream the butter, yogurt, and sugar together using a fork.

4. Beat in the egg. Add milk and vanilla and stir until well blended.

5. In a large mixing bowl, combine flour, baking powder, and cinnamon. Stir until evenly combined.

6. Create a well in the middle of the dry ingredients and gently pour the wet ingredients into the well. Stir ingredients into a batter.

7. Gently fold in the rhubarb until evenly mixed into the batter. Spread batter into the prepared cake pan. Top evenly with streusel.

8. Bake for 40 minutes; let cool for 20 minutes prior to serving.

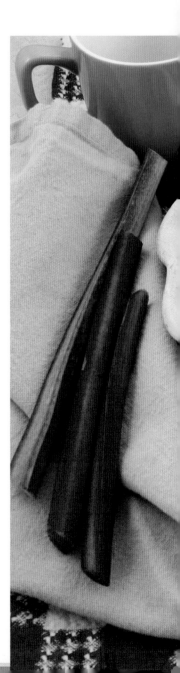

## NUTRITION INFORMATION

Serving size: 1/12 recipe

Per serving: 210 calories, 8 g total fat, 2.5 g saturated fat, 25 mg cholesterol, 33g carbohydrates, 3 g fiber, 22 g sugars, 4 g protein, and 105 mg sodium.

CACFP: serve with 1/2 cup fluid milk, 1/2 cup fruit or vegetable, 1/2 ounce cheese, or 2 ounces yogurt to meet the snack requirement.

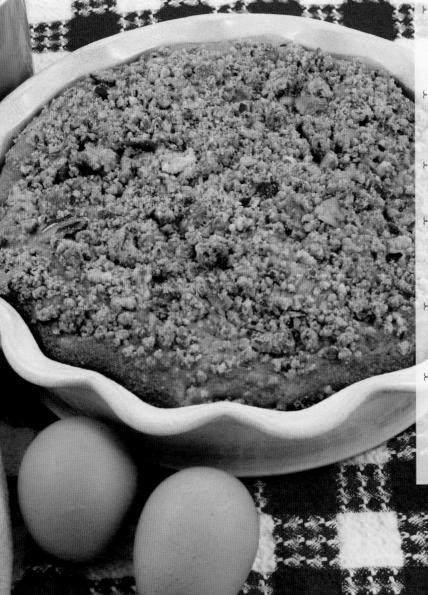

- The word *rhubarb* comes from the Latin *rhabarbarum* "root of the barbarians" because the Romans believed people who ate it to be barbaric in nature.

- Although rhubarb is typically considered a fruit, it is really a vegetable.

- Only two vegetables (rhubarb and asparagus) are perennials, meaning they can produce on their own for several growing seasons.

- Rhubarb is often used as a pie filling. Rhubarb is almost always sweetened with sugar to help balance its natural tartness.

- Rhubarb comes in many varieties and colors, but commercially grown rhubarb is generally red.

- Rhubarb is usually available from late winter to early spring, but can be found in limited quantities at other times of the year.

- Color is the main indicator of quality in rhubarb. Rhubarb should be red in color and should be free from any defects.

- Rhubarb is readily available in the spring. Try freezing it to make it last throughout the year by following these simple steps: wash and trim it, boil for one minute, place in a sealed container and freeze.

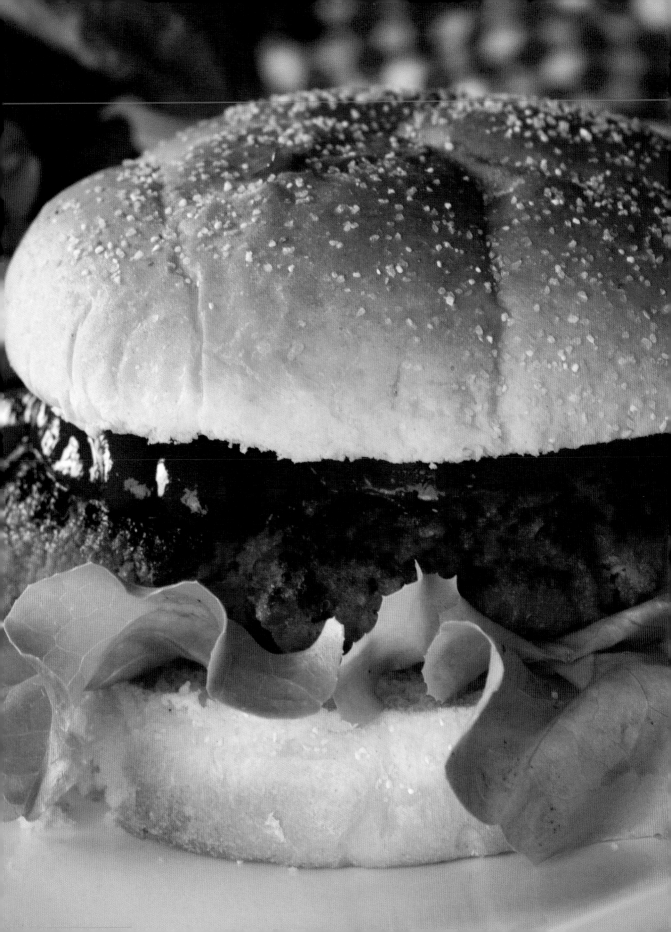

# Turkey Burgers

Estimated preparation and cooking time: 25 minutes

## INGREDIENTS

½ cup dry bread crumbs

6 tablespoons ketchup

⅛ teaspoon ground pepper

1½ pounds lean ground turkey

2 teaspoons canola oil (if frying burgers on the stove)

## PROCEDURE

1. In medium bowl, combine all ingredients except vegetable oil. With fork, mix ingredients until blended. Do not overwork, or burgers will be tough.

2. Divide mixture into 10 servings. Wet hands with water and shape each mound into flat circle. Place burgers on plate.

3. If frying burgers on stove, add vegetable oil to frying pan. Set on medium-low. Heat pan with oil 1 minute. Place burgers in pan; cook until bottoms are brown (about 5 minutes), flip over and cook 5–7 minutes to internal temperature of 165°F.

4. If grilling burgers: Grill on oiled rack 5–7 minutes on each side to internal temperature of 165°F.

Yield: 10 servings

## NUTRITION INFORMATION

Serving size: 1 burger

Per serving: 140 calories, 7 g total fat, 1½ g saturated fat, 55 mg cholesterol, 6 g carbohydrates, 0 g fiber, 2 g sugars, 13 g protein, and 200 mg sodium

CACFP: Serve on a whole grain roll with ¼ cup Sweet Potato Wedges, ¼ cup fruit, such as melon or peaches, and ¾ cup fluid milk.

⸎ Ground turkey is a healthy substitute for ground beef. It's low in saturated fat and high in protein.

⸎ As with any uncooked meat, raw turkey should not be handled by young children. Be sure to wash and sanitize any bowls, plates, and utensils that come in contact with it, and wash hands thoroughly.

⸎ Benjamin Franklin proposed the turkey, not the bald eagle, as the national bird of the United States. Comparing the eagle to the turkey, Franklin wrote, "The turkey is in comparison a much more respectable bird, and withal a true original native of America."

⸎ While most domesticated turkeys can't fly, wild ones can fly as fast as 55 mph.

⸎ Contrary to popular belief, eating turkey doesn't make you sleepy. It's eating a lot of carbohydrates at a big holiday meal that causes drowsiness.

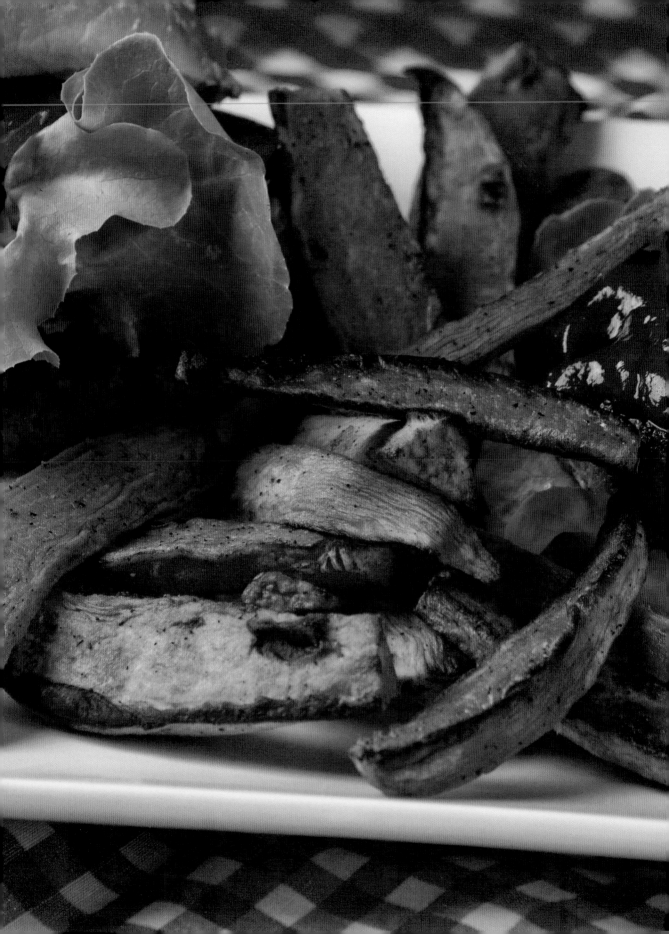

# Sweet Potato Wedges

Estimated preparation and cooking time: 40 minutes

## INGREDIENTS

2 pounds sweet potatoes (about 2 large sweet potatoes)

1 tablespoon canola oil

1/8 teaspoon salt

1/8 teaspoon pepper

Nonstick cooking spray

## PROCEDURE

1. Preheat oven to 400°F. Lightly coat two large baking sheets with nonstick cooking spray.

2. Peel sweet potatoes.

3. Cut sweet potatoes crosswise into 1/4-inch thick slices. Then cut each slice into quarters.

4. Place sweet potato pieces in large mixing bowl; add canola oil, salt, and pepper. Toss well to coat.

5. Spread potatoes on baking sheets in single layer.

6. Bake 20–25 minutes, flipping after 10 minutes.

7. Cool slightly and serve.

Yield: 18 servings

## NUTRITION INFORMATION

Serving size: 1/4 cup

Per serving: 40 calories, 1 g total fat, 0 g saturated fat, 10 mg cholesterol, 8 g carbohydrates, 1 g fiber, 3 g sugars, 1 g protein, and 30 mg sodium

CACFP: Sweet Potato Wedges meet half of the vegetable/fruit requirement for lunch when 1/4 cup is served per child.

⚘ Serve these delicious pseudo-fries with our turkey burgers for a healthy twist to a favorite meal—sweet potatoes are significantly higher in many vitamins and minerals than white potatoes.

⚘ As early as 750 BCE, sweet potatoes were grown in what is now Peru.

⚘ Yams and sweet potatoes are not the same thing. In fact, they aren't even related botanically. Several species of yams are actually toxic if eaten fresh.

⚘ This recipe makes about eighteen 1/4-cup servings. If you want to serve it for snack, increasing the amount of raw sweet potato to 2 1/2–3 pounds will give you enough for ten 1/2-cup servings.

# Squash & Apple Soup

Estimated preparation and cooking time: 1 hour and 25 minutes

## INGREDIENTS

3 cups cooked butternut squash

2 tablespoons canola oil

½ cup chopped onion

1 medium clove garlic, crushed or minced

1 teaspoon salt

½ teaspoon ground cumin

½ teaspoon ground coriander

½ teaspoon ground cinnamon

¾ teaspoon ground ginger

¼ teaspoon dry mustard

2 medium Granny Smith apples, peeled and chopped

2½ cups water

1 cup orange juice

## PROCEDURE

1. **Cut squash in half lengthwise. Do not scoop out seeds. Place cut side down in baking dish with 1 inch water; bake at 400°F 30–40 minutes or until flesh is soft. Allow squash to cool thoroughly. Scoop out seeds and discard. Measure out 3 cups cooked squash.**

2. **Heat canola oil in skillet; add onion, garlic, salt, and spices. Sauté until onion is very soft. Add apple, cover, and cook, stirring frequently, 10 minutes, or until apple is soft (you may need to add a little water to prevent sticking).**

3. **Place onion and apple mixture, squash, water, and orange juice in food processor or blender and purée until smooth.**

4. **Reheat gently; serve with Multigrain Rolls (page 140) or Harvest Muffins (page 59).**

Yield: 10 servings

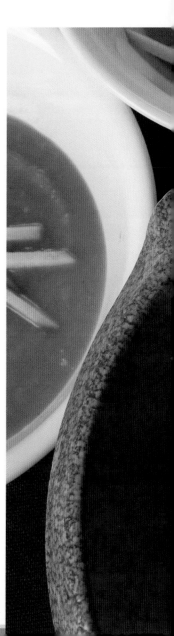

## NUTRITION INFORMATION

Serving size: ¹/₁₀ recipe

Per serving: 80 calories, 3 g total fat, 0 g saturated fat, 0 mg cholesterol, 15 g carbohydrates, 3 g dietary fiber, 6 g sugars, 1 g protein, and 260 mg sodium

CACFP: A serving of Squash and Apple Soup meets the fruit/vegetable requirement for lunch. Serve with ¾ cup fluid milk, 1½ ounces meat or meat alternate, and a Multigrain Roll.

⚶ When it's time to pick apples and squash, you know autumn is here. This soup is a great way to enjoy both of these foods while celebrating the season.

⚶ Butternut squash can also be cooked in a microwave or steamed. You can also use frozen squash, cooked according to package directions, or canned squash.

⚶ Butternut squash is a good source of vitamin A, vitamin C, potassium, folic acid, calcium, and magnesium.

⚶ In Australia, butternut squash is called *butternut pumpkin*.

⚶ Indigenous populations in South America cultivated different varieties of squash between 8,000 and 10,000 years ago.

⚶ Butternut squash is a winter squash. Other winter squashes include buttercup, acorn, Hubbard, delicata, and spaghetti squash.

⚶ The spice cumin comes from the seed of a plant related to the carrot. It is popular in Asian, Indian, Mexican, and North African cooking. Other spices in this family include anise, caraway, coriander, and celery seed.

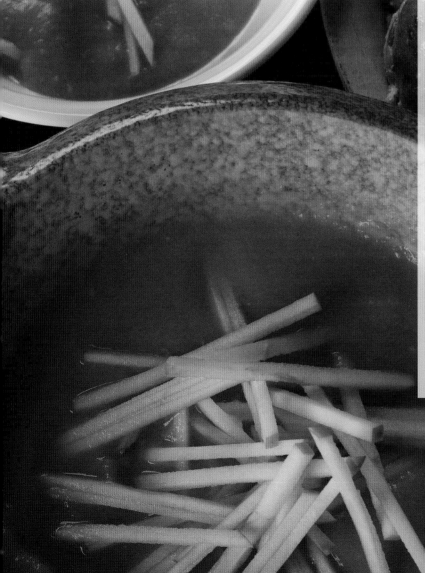

# Multigrain Rolls

Estimated preparation and cooking time: 2 hours and 45 minutes

## INGREDIENTS

¼ cup bulgur wheat

¼ cup rolled oats

2 tablespoons sesame seeds

2 tablespoons millet

2 tablespoons sunflower seeds

1½ cups boiling water

2 tablespoons canola oil

2 tablespoons brown sugar

½ teaspoon salt

2 teaspoons yeast

2–4 tablespoons warm water

3½ cups white whole wheat flour

Nonstick cooking spray

## PROCEDURE

1. Measure bulgur, oats, sesame seeds, millet, and sunflower seeds into large bowl. Add 1½ cups boiling water, stir, and let sit 20 minutes.

2. After 20 minutes, add oil, brown sugar, yeast, salt, and 2 tablespoons water to grain mixture. Mix together. Gradually add flour, mixing until dough becomes too stiff to stir.

3. Flour clean tabletop or large cutting board; turn dough onto it. Knead dough, mixing in remaining flour, 5–10 minutes or until dough is smooth and elastic (you may need to add 1–2 tablespoons water if dough is too dry).

4. Lightly coat large bowl with nonstick cooking spray; add dough, turning until all its surfaces are lightly oiled. Cover bowl with plastic wrap; leave in warm place for 1 hour or until dough has doubled in size.

5. Punch down dough and turn out onto lightly floured surface. Divide into 20 pieces; roll each piece to form firm ball.

6. Coat 9 x 13-inch baking pan with nonstick cooking spray. Place balls of dough in pan. (It's okay if sides of rolls touch.) Cover pan with plastic wrap; leave in warm place 30 minutes. While rolls rise, preheat oven to 400°F.

7. Bake rolls 25 minutes or until golden. Cool and serve.

Yield: 20 rolls

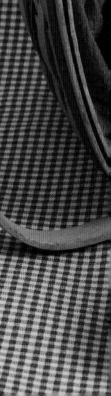

## NUTRITION INFORMATION

Serving size: 1 roll

Per serving: 130 calories, 3 g total fat, 0 g saturated fat, 0 mg cholesterol, 21 g carbohydrates, 3 g dietary fiber, 1 g sugars, 4 g protein, and 60 mg sodium

CACFP: ½ of a Multigrain Roll meets the grain requirement for breakfast, lunch, or snack.

⨞ You can also use this recipe to make a loaf of bread. Follow steps 1 through 5. Instead of dividing the dough into 20 pieces, shape and place it in an oiled bread pan, let rise 20–30 minutes, and bake at 400°F 25–30 minutes.

⨞ Until recently, you were more likely to find millet in birdseed mixes than food for humans in the United States, but it's a whole grain (technically a seed) that has been grown and eaten in Africa and Asia for thousands of years. Millet is high in protein and manganese. Many grocery stores now carry millet in their bulk foods or health food sections.

⨞ Sesame seeds are a very versatile food—they're used as a spice, in candy, noodle, and vegetable dishes, ground into tahini, and pressed for their oil.

⨞ The phrase "Open sesame!" is thought to stem from the tendency of sesame seeds to pop loudly from their pods when they ripen.

⨞ Sunflower seeds, which are rich in vitamin E and antioxidants, are also grown for their oil and eaten whole in a variety of foods. Sunflower butter is a popular spread for crackers and sandwiches. It is a good option if your school is nut free.

⨞ Mature sunflowers always face to the east. The plants can grow to more than 20 feet tall, and the flowers can be more than 2 feet across.

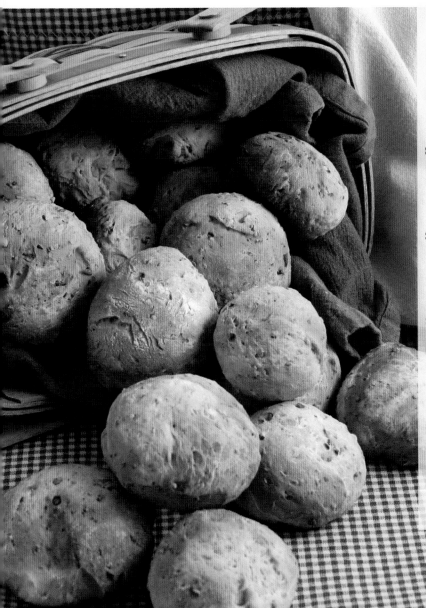

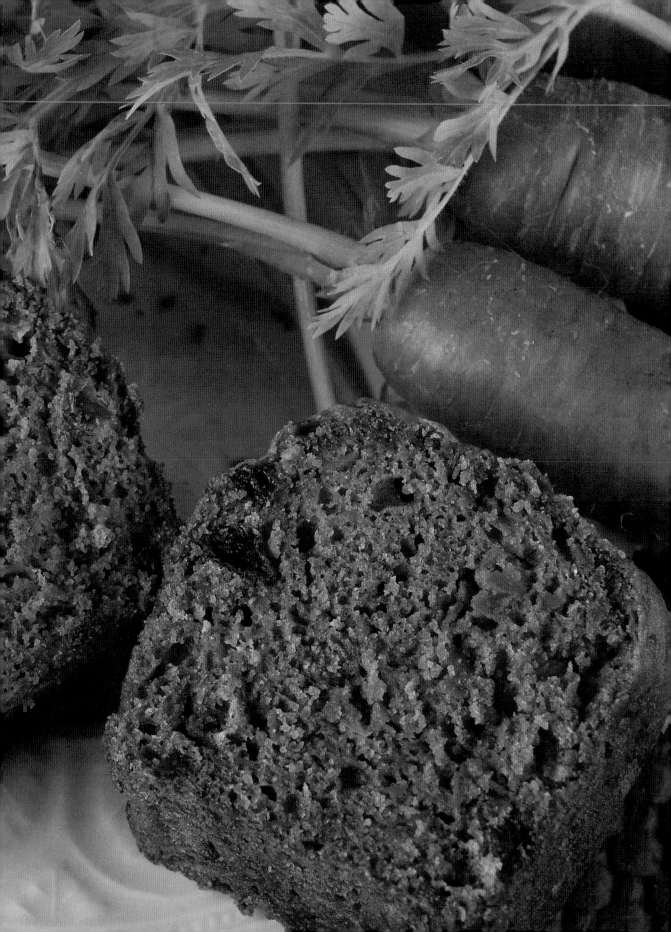

# Carrot Cake

Estimated preparation and cooking time: 1 hour

## INGREDIENTS

1½ cups packed finely shredded carrots

2 large eggs

¾ cup pure maple syrup

¼ cup orange juice

½ cup golden or regular raisins

5 tablespoons canola oil

1½ cups white whole wheat flour

1 teaspoon baking powder

1 teaspoon baking soda

2 teaspoon ground cinnamon

½ teaspoon salt

Nonstick cooking spray

## PROCEDURE

1. Preheat oven to 350°F.

2. Lightly spray 9 x 13-inch baking pan with nonstick cooking spray.

3. Wash carrots and shred in food processor or with grater.

4. In medium bowl, whisk together eggs and maple syrup.

5. Stir in shredded carrots, orange juice, raisins, and canola oil.

6. In large bowl, combine flour, baking powder, baking soda, cinnamon, and salt.

7. Create well in middle of dry ingredients. Slowly add liquid ingredients. Mix only until dry ingredients are moistened. Do not overmix.

8. Spoon batter into prepared pan; bake 40 minutes at 350°F or until toothpick comes out clean when inserted into center of cake.

9. Allow cake to cool before serving. Cut into 12 portions.

Yield: 12 servings

- It takes about 4½ pounds of grapes to make 1 pound of raisins.

- Grapes are a good source of vitamin C and vitamin K and are very low in saturated fats. But raisins also are very high in sugars.

- Even in this age of modern food production, most raisins are still made by drying the grapes on trays under the sun.

- Ancient Romans used raisins as medicine, prizes, and currency.

- In 1492 Christopher Columbus sailed to the New World with raisins on board his ships.

## NUTRITION INFORMATION

Serving size: ¹/₁₂ recipe

Per serving: 200 calories, 7 g total fat, ½ g saturated fat, 30 mg cholesterol, 33 g carbohydrates, 3 g dietary fiber, 16 g sugars, 3 g protein, and 260 mg sodium

CACFP: Serve with ½ cup fluid milk, 6 tablespoons fruit or vegetable, or 2 ounces yogurt to meet the snack requirement.

# Butternut Squash Cake

Estimated preparation and cooking time: 2 days
(45 minutes the day before and 1 hour and 10 minutes the day of serving)

## INGREDIENTS

2 cups cooked, puréed butternut squash

¾ cup sugar

½ cup canola oil

4 eggs

1 teaspoon vanilla extract

2 cups white whole wheat flour

2 teaspoons baking powder

1 teaspoon baking soda

1 teaspoon cinnamon

½ teaspoon salt

Nonstick cooking spray

## PROCEDURE

1. Cut squash in half lengthwise. Do not scoop out seeds. Place cut side down in baking dish with 1 inch of water; bake at 400°F 30–40 minutes or until flesh is soft. Allow squash to cool thoroughly. Scoop out seeds and discard. Scoop out and measure 2 cups cooked squash. Mash well with fork or potato masher.

2. Turn oven down to 350° F.

3. Spray 9 x 13-inch baking pan with nonstick cooking spray.

4. In large bowl, stir together squash, sugar, oil, eggs, and vanilla.

5. In medium bowl, combine flour, baking powder, baking soda, cinnamon, and salt.

6. Add flour mixture to squash mixture. Stir only until flour mixture is fully moistened. Do not overmix.

7. Spread batter into prepared pan; bake 40 minutes or until toothpick comes out clean when inserted into center of cake.

Yield: 18 servings

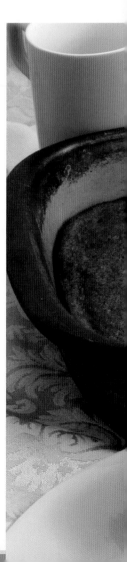

## NUTRITION INFORMATION

Serving size: $1/18$ recipe

Per serving: 170 calories, 7 g total fat, ½ g saturated fat, 40 mg cholesterol, 22 g carbohydrates, 3 g dietary fiber, 9 g sugars, 4 g protein, and 200 mg sodium

CACFP: Serve with ½ cup fluid milk, ½ cup fruit or vegetable, or 2 ounces yogurt to meet the snack requirement.

⸾ Canned (or frozen) squash or pumpkin can be used in place of fresh butternut squash.

⸾ People don't usually think of vegetables as ingredients for cakes, but puréed squash or shredded carrots (zucchini too) add moisture and nutrients, making this treat food healthy and tasty.

⸾ Using a healthy oil such as canola instead of a solid fat also increases moistness while improving the nutritional value of a cake.

⸾ The world's largest birthday cake weighed 130,000 pounds and measured 102 x 52 feet (and was 20 inches tall).

⸾ Birthdays are celebrated with different foods around the world. Depending on where you live, you might have pie, noodles, rice and beans, fried plantains, or fufu (a mixture of yam and cassava).

# NINE

⌁

## ORIGINAL
## EARLY SPROUTS
## RECIPES

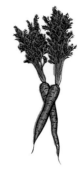

In this chapter we share with you many of the recipes from our first Early Sprouts book. These recipes were designed to be cooked with young children and are therefore quite simple to prepare. The recipes were also created to provide multiple exposures to the target vegetables featured in the Early Sprouts program, lend themselves to being easily packed in a family recipe kit, and contain readily available and affordable ingredients. And much like the other recipes in this book, the recipes feature fruits/vegetables, whole grains, healthy fats, and low-fat dairy. We hope you enjoy them and take the opportunity to prepare them with the preschoolers in your life.

# Cherry Tomatoes with Honey Mustard Dip

Estimated preparation and cooking time: 20 minutes

## INGREDIENTS

1 pint of cherry tomatoes (20–24 tomatoes)

½ cup of low-fat or nonfat plain yogurt

2 teaspoons spicy brown mustard

2 teaspoons honey

## PROCEDURE

1. Wash cherry tomatoes, slice in half, and set aside.

2. Measure and place yogurt, mustard, and honey in medium bowl.

3. Stir until well mixed and smooth.

4. Pour dressing into small dipping cups or bowls.

5. Enjoy cherry tomatoes dipped in honey mustard dressing.

Yield: 8 servings

## NUTRITION INFORMATION

Serving size: ⅛ recipe

Per serving: 22 calories, <1 g total fat, 0 g saturated fat, 1 mg cholesterol, 4 g carbohydrates, .5 g fiber, 3 g sugars, and 22 mg sodium

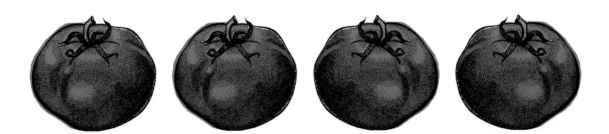

# Chinese-Style Green Beans

Estimated preparation and cooking time: 25 minutes

## INGREDIENTS

1 pound green beans

4 teaspoons unsalted butter

4 teaspoons low sodium tamari

2 teaspoons fresh lemon juice
  (¼ lemon squeezed)

## PROCEDURE

1. In nonstick skillet, melt butter over low heat on stovetop. Place medium pot of water on another burner and bring it to a boil.

2. Clean green beans, remove stems, and snap in half.

3. When butter has melted, remove from heat and use wooden spoon to stir in tamari and lemon juice. Set aside.

4. Add green beans to boiling water and boil 5 minutes, or until tender.

5. Turn off heat and drain green beans in colander.

6. Add green beans to butter/tamari mixture and gently toss to combine

Yield: 8 servings

## NUTRITION INFORMATION

Serving size: ⅛ recipe

Per serving: 35 calories, 2 g total fat, 1 g saturated fat, 5 mg cholesterol, 4 g carbohydrates, 2 g fiber, 1 g sugar, and 154 mg sodium

# Bell Pepper–Couscous Castles

Estimated preparation and cooking time: 25 minutes

## INGREDIENTS

1 diced bell pepper

½ cup (thawed) frozen corn

Vegetable oil

2 cups vegetable broth

2 cups whole wheat couscous

Small pinch paprika (optional)

Ice cubes

## PROCEDURE

1. Clean bell pepper, remove seeds, and dice into small pieces.

2. Coat skillet with small amount of vegetable oil. Add diced bell pepper and corn to skillet. Raise heat to medium-high and sauté vegetables until tender.

3. Add vegetable broth and couscous to skillet. Cook, stirring continuously, about 5 minutes or until broth has been absorbed. Remove skillet from heat, cover, and let sit another minute or two.

4. Transfer couscous and vegetables to large mixing bowl and stir. Add ice cubes, one at a time, while stirring, until mixture cools enough to handle.

5. Use ⅓ cup measuring cup to pack couscous mixture, and then turn it upside down onto small plate to create castles. Makes about 8 castles.

6. If desired, lightly sprinkle castles with paprika.

Yield: 8 servings

## NUTRITION INFORMATION

Serving size: ⅛ recipe

Per serving: 66 calories, 1 g total fat, 0 g saturated fat, 0 mg cholesterol, 13 g carbohydrates, 2 g fiber, 1 g sugar, and 118 mg sodium

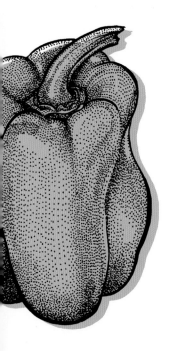

# Cheddar & Chard Quesadillas

Estimated preparation and cooking time: 35 minutes

## INGREDIENTS

⅔ pound Swiss chard

1 cup shredded cheddar cheese

4 whole wheat tortillas or wraps

Nonstick cooking spray

Optional: low-fat sour cream, salsa, and/or guacamole

## PROCEDURE

1. Preheat oven to 400°F.

2. Wash Swiss chard and remove stems.

3. Cut or tear chard into 2-inch pieces.

4. Heat saucepan sprayed lightly with nonstick cooking spray. Add chard to pan and cook just until limp. Set aside to cool.

5. Lightly coat baking sheet with nonstick cooking spray.

6. Place 2 tortillas on baking sheet. Sprinkle shredded cheese evenly over each tortilla. Evenly spread chard on top of cheese. Cover with remaining tortillas.

7. Lightly mist top of tortillas with a bit more nonstick cooking spray. Bake in preheated oven for approximately 15 minutes.

8. Allow to cool and then cut into fourths. Transfer to serving plate. Serve with low-fat sour cream, salsa, and/or guacamole, if desired.

Yield: 8 servings

## NUTRITION INFORMATION

Serving size: ¼ quesadilla

Per serving: 134 calories, 6 g total fat, 3 g saturated fat, 15 mg cholesterol, 13 g carbohydrates, 2 g fiber, 1 g sugar, and 250 mg sodium

# Carrot-Oatmeal Cookies

Estimated preparation and cooking time: 40 minutes

## INGREDIENTS

2 cups (6 ounces) shredded carrots, about 3 medium-large carrots

½ cup canola or vegetable oil

½ cup sugar

1 teaspoon vanilla

2 large eggs

2 cups white whole wheat flour

1 cup rolled oats

1 teaspoon ground cinnamon

1 teaspoon baking powder

½ teaspoon salt

Nonstick cooking spray or 2–4 teaspoons vegetable oil

## PROCEDURE

1. Preheat oven to 375°F.

2. Spray cookie sheet with nonstick cooking spray or lightly coat with vegetable oil.

3. Wash carrots and grate using food processor or hand grater.

4. In medium bowl, use fork to beat oil and sugar together until well combined.

5. In small bowl, beat eggs using fork. Add to oil mixture. Add carrots and vanilla.

6. In large bowl, combine flour, oats, cinnamon, baking powder, and salt. Stir until evenly combined.

7. Create well in middle of dry ingredients. Slowly add oil mixture. Stir until wet and dry ingredients are evenly combined.

8. Using large dinner spoon, drop batter onto cookie sheet, leaving 2-inch space between cookies.

9. Bake 15 to 18 minutes or until golden brown.

10. Allow cookies to cool before serving.

Yield: 8 servings

## NUTRITION INFORMATION

Serving size: 1 cookie

Per serving: 120 calories, 5 g total fat, 1 g saturated fat, 15 mg cholesterol, 16 g carbohydrates, 2 g fiber, 4 g sugar, and 76 mg sodium

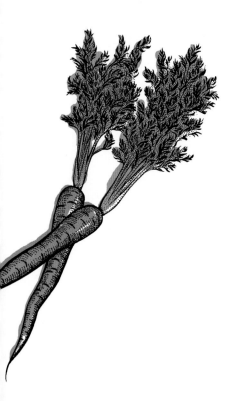

# Butternut Squash Pancakes

Estimated preparation and cooking time: 30 minutes

## INGREDIENTS

1½ cups cooked butternut squash

1 cup white whole wheat flour

1 teaspoon cinnamon

2 teaspoons brown sugar

½ teaspoon salt

2 teaspoons baking powder

1 tablespoon canola or other vegetable oil

1½ cups milk

2 eggs

Nonstick cooking spray

Optional: Maple syrup

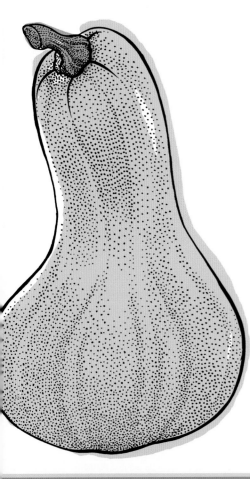

## PROCEDURE

1. Preheat oven to 400°F. Fill baking dish with about an inch of water.

2. Cut butternut squash in half from top to bottom. Do not scoop out seeds. Place squash cut side down in baking dish with water and bake 30–40 minutes or until flesh is soft.

3. Allow squash to cool thoroughly. Scoop seeds out of squash and discard. Scoop out cooked squash and measure 1½ cups.

4. Mix in blender until well combined: squash, flour, cinnamon, brown sugar, salt, baking powder, canola oil, egg, and milk.

5. Lightly coat griddle or large skillet with nonstick cooking spray.

6. Pour batter onto griddle in silver-dollar-sized pancakes.

7. When batter is fairly covered with bubbles, flip pancakes. Cook until both sides are golden brown.

8. Allow pancakes to cool and serve with warm maple syrup, if desired.

Yield: 8 servings

## NUTRITION INFORMATION

Serving size: 2 pancakes

Per serving: 140 calories, 4 g total fat, 1 g saturated fat, 40 mg cholesterol, 20 g carbohydrates, 3.5 g fiber, 4 g sugar, and 283 mg sodium

# Pasta with Garlic-Parmesan Tomato Sauce

Estimated preparation and cooking time: 25 minutes

## INGREDIENTS

½ pound whole wheat pasta

3 cups cherry tomatoes

2 cloves fresh garlic

¼ heaping cup grated Parmesan cheese

¼ cup low-sodium vegetable broth

1 tablespoon olive or other vegetable oil

## PROCEDURE

1. Bring approximately 6 cups water to rolling boil over high heat.

2. Meanwhile, gently rinse cherry tomatoes. Cut tomatoes in half.

3. Remove outer skin from garlic cloves. Crush cloves in garlic press or use knife to finely mince.

4. Add pasta to boiling water and cook approximately 10 minutes.

5. Add tomatoes and broth to blender. Use pulse mechanism to coarsely chop and incorporate ingredients.

6. When pasta has finished cooking, remove from heat, drain, and rinse with cold water to stop it from cooking.

7. Heat olive oil in skillet on medium-high heat. When oil is hot, add minced garlic, cook for 30 seconds, and then add tomato sauce from blender. Reduce heat and simmer about 5 minutes to cook off excess liquid.

8. Add cooked pasta to skillet and stir to coat with sauce. Heat another minute or two; then remove from heat and transfer to serving dish.

9. Sprinkle cheese on top of pasta.

Yield: 8 servings

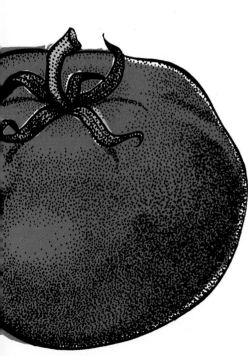

## NUTRITION INFORMATION

Serving size: ⅛ recipe

Per serving: 140 calories, 3 g total fat, 1 g saturated fat, 0 mg cholesterol, 24 g carbohydrates, 3 g fiber, 2 g sugar, and 75 mg sodium

# Green Bean Wontons with Dipping Sauce

Estimated preparation and cooking time: 30 minutes

## INGREDIENTS

2 cups green beans

16 wonton wrappers

¼ cup rice vinegar

2 tablespoons low-sodium, wheat-free tamari

2 teaspoons honey

2 tablespoons canola or vegetable oil

## PROCEDURE

1. Clean green beans and remove stems. Shred green beans using food processor or chop finely with knife.

2. Heat oil in nonstick skillet over medium to high heat. Sauté shredded green beans until tender. Allow to cool.

3. To create green bean wonton, take one wonton wrapper, place ½ tablespoon shredded green beans in center, wet all sides with water using finger, and fold wonton into triangle. Press edges together. Repeat until you've made all 16 wontons, or as many as you want.

4. Heat a small amount of oil in nonstick skillet.

5. Sauté wontons 2–3 minutes per side or until slightly golden.

6. While wontons are cooking, prepare dipping sauce by mixing tamari, rice vinegar, and honey in small bowl.

7. Remove wontons from pan. As soon as wontons reach safe eating temperature, serve with dipping sauce.

Yield: 8 servings

## NUTRITION INFORMATION

Serving size: ⅛ recipe

Per serving: 45 calories, 2 g total fat, 0 g saturated fat, 0 mg cholesterol, 6 g carbohydrates, 1 g fiber, 1 g sugar, and 170 mg sodium

# Confetti Corn Muffins

Estimated preparation and cooking time: 40 minutes

## INGREDIENTS

½ bell pepper

1 cup cornmeal (fine milled)

½ cup white whole wheat flour

¼ teaspoon salt

1 teaspoon baking powder

½ teaspoon baking soda

1½ cups low-fat plain yogurt

3 tablespoons honey

2 large eggs

3 tablespoons canola or other vegetable oil

⅔ cup shredded sharp cheddar cheese

Nonstick cooking spray or vegetable oil

## PROCEDURE

1. Preheat oven to 400°F.

2. Coat muffin tins with nonstick cooking spray or wipe tins with paper towel coated with vegetable oil.

3. Clean bell pepper and remove seeds. Finely dice pepper. Set diced pepper aside.

4. Place in large mixing bowl: cornmeal, flour, salt, baking powder, and baking soda.

5. Whisk together in medium mixing bowl: yogurt, honey, eggs, and oil.

6. Create well in center of dry mixture. Fill with wet ingredients. Gently stir until all ingredients are incorporated. Do not overstir.

7. Gently fold half of shredded cheddar cheese into batter.

8. Fill muffin tins ¾ full. Sprinkle diced bell peppers on top of batter, followed by remaining cheddar cheese.

9. Bake 15–20 minutes or until golden brown. (Mini muffins bake faster than regular muffins.) Allow to cool slightly before removing from pan. Enjoy!

Yield: 12 muffins or 24 mini muffins

## NUTRITION INFORMATION

Serving size: 1 muffin or 2 mini muffins

Per serving: 166 calories, 7 g total fat, 2 g saturated fat, 40 mg cholesterol, 20 g carbohydrates, 2 g fiber, 7 g sugar, and 200 mg sodium

# Pita Pocket Pizzas

Estimated preparation and cooking time: 20 minutes

## INGREDIENTS

8 to 12 Swiss chard leaves

1 tablespoon plus 1 teaspoon olive or other vegetable oil

½ cup tomato sauce

¼ teaspoon garlic powder and ¼ teaspoon Italian spices (no salt added)

4 whole wheat pita bread rounds

⅔ cup shredded mozzarella cheese

## PROCEDURE

1. Preheat oven to 400°F.

2. Wash and dry chard. Stack washed chard leaves with all stems facing same direction. Cut triangle shape around stems, separating leaves from stems. Stack leaves again and chop finely.

3. Heat oil in skillet for about 1 minute. Add chard and cook, stirring occasionally, 2 minutes.

4. Remove skillet from heat. Carefully add tomato sauce to pan, stirring gently until leaves and sauce are combined.

5. Add garlic powder and spices; stir.

6. Lay pita bread on large baking sheet.

7. Spread approximately 2 tablespoons sauce on each pita round. Sprinkle cheese on top of each pita.

8. Bake approximately 7–10 minutes or until cheese is bubbly.

9. Remove from oven. Cut each round into 4 slices.

Yield: 8 servings

## NUTRITION INFORMATION

Serving size: 2 slices

Per serving: 70 calories, 2.5 g total fat, 2 g saturated fat, 5 mg cholesterol, 10 g carbohydrates, 2 g fiber, 1 g sugar, and 220 mg sodium

# Honey-Glazed Carrots

Estimated preparation and cooking time: 40–45 minutes

## INGREDIENTS

1½ pounds carrots

2 tablespoons butter

3 teaspoons low-sodium tamari

3 tablespoons honey

## PROCEDURE

1. Wash and peel carrots.

2. Steam carrots until just tender. Rinse in strainer under cold water to cool.

3. Cut carrots into bite-sized pieces.

4. Place butter and tamari in saucepan and cook over medium-low heat.

5. Add garlic powder and spices; stir.

6. Once butter is melted, add honey.

7. Stir in steamed carrots and mix until all carrots are glazed.

Yield: 8 servings

## NUTRITION INFORMATION

Serving size: ⅛ recipe

Per serving: 65 calories, 2.5 g total fat, 1.5 g saturated fat, 6 mg cholesterol, 11 g carbohydrates, 2 g fiber, 8 g sugar, and 150 mg sodium

# English Muffin Pizzas with Homemade Sauce

Estimated preparation and cooking time: 35 minutes

## INGREDIENTS

2 cups cherry tomatoes, washed (about 20 tomatoes)

3 teaspoons olive or other vegetable oil

4 whole wheat English muffins

1½ cups shredded part-skim mozzarella cheese

1 teaspoon sugar

## PROCEDURE

1. Preheat oven to 400°F.

2. Rinse cherry tomatoes and cut in half.

3. Heat 3 teaspoons oil in skillet over medium heat. Add halved tomatoes to skillet; sprinkle with sugar. Sauté 5–6 minutes.

4. Transfer contents of skillet to blender or food processor and purée. Pour puréed tomato sauce into shallow bowl.

5. Split English muffins in half and place on ungreased baking sheet.

6. To assemble each pizza, spoon 2 tablespoons sauce onto English muffin "crusts," spreading with back of spoon. Cover each pizza with cheese.

7. Bake pizzas 10–15 minutes or until cheese is bubbly and just beginning to brown.

8. Allow pizzas to cool slightly and cut in halves or quarters. Transfer to serving platter, serve, and enjoy!

Yield: 8 servings

## NUTRITION INFORMATION

Serving size: ½ muffin

Per serving: 140 calories, 6 g total fat, 2.5 g saturated fat, 16 mg cholesterol, 16 g carbohydrates, 3 g fiber, 4 g sugar, and 289 mg sodium

# Sesame Seed Green Beans

Estimated preparation and cooking time: 30 minutes

## INGREDIENTS

⅔ to 1 pound fresh green beans

¼ cup sesame seeds for sprinkling

Salt and pepper to taste

2 teaspoons olive oil

## PROCEDURE

1. Wash green beans and trim off ends. Snap beans in half.

2. Pour oil into skillet and warm over medium heat.

3. Add green beans to skillet and sauté 5–8 minutes or until tender.

4. Season beans with salt and pepper.

5. Serve beans in small bowls and enjoy! Invite your family to sprinkle sesame seeds on their green beans if they like.

Yield: 8 servings

## NUTRITION INFORMATION

Serving size: ⅛ recipe

Per serving: 40 calories, 2.5 g total fat, 0 g saturated fat, 0 mg cholesterol, 4 g carbohydrates, 2 g fiber, 1 g sugar, and 0 mg sodium

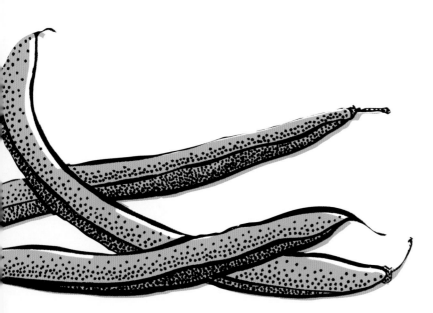

# Lemony Swiss Chard Pasta

Estimated preparation and cooking time: 40 minutes

## INGREDIENTS

⅔ pound whole wheat pasta

6 leaves Swiss chard

1 small or medium lemon

2 pinches sea salt and pepper

1 tablespoon plus 1 teaspoon
   olive oil or other vegetable oil

10 ounces feta cheese

## PROCEDURE

1. Bring pot of water to boil. Add pasta to pot and cook 10 minutes or until al dente, stirring occasionally.

2. Meanwhile, wash chard, remove stems, and cut chard into small, ⅓–½-inch pieces.

3. Squeeze lemon juice into large bowl.

4. In large bowl, whisk together lemon juice, salt, pepper, and olive oil.

5. Chop feta cheese into small pieces.

6. When pasta is cooked, drain, rinse, and add pasta, chard, and feta to bowl of dressing.

7. Toss until well combined.

Yield: 8 servings

## NUTRITION INFORMATION

Serving size: ⅛ recipe

Per serving: 210 calories, 7 g total fat, 3 g saturated fat, 15 mg cholesterol, 32 g carbohydrates, 4 g fiber, 1 g sugar, and 350 mg sodium

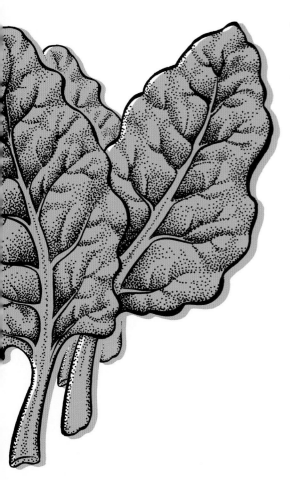

# Carrot Sticks with Vanilla Dip

Estimated preparation time: 15 minutes

## INGREDIENTS

1 cup low-fat vanilla yogurt

½ teaspoon cinnamon

3 teaspoons honey

40–50 baby carrots

## PROCEDURE

1. Measure yogurt, honey, and cinnamon into a small bowl.

2. Mix together and serve it as a dip with the carrots.

Yield: 8 servings

## NUTRITION INFORMATION

Serving size: ⅛ recipe

Per serving: 35 calories, 0 g total fat, 0 g saturated fat, 0 mg cholesterol, 7 g carbohydrates, 1 g fiber, 6 g sugar, and 40 mg sodium

# Tomato & Cheese Quesadillas

Estimated preparation and cooking time: 35 minutes

## INGREDIENTS

2 medium tomatoes

1⅓ cups shredded Monterey Jack cheese

4 whole wheat tortillas or wraps

Nonstick cooking spray

Optional: salsa, low-fat sour cream, and/or guacamole

## PROCEDURE

1. Preheat oven to 400°F.

2. Wash tomato and cut into thick slices.

3. Lightly coat baking sheet with nonstick cooking spray.

4. Place two tortillas on baking sheet. Sprinkle shredded cheese evenly over two tortillas. Top cheese with single layer of tomato slices. Cover topped tortillas with remaining tortillas.

5. Lightly mist top of each tortilla with vegetable oil spray. Bake in oven for approximately 15 minutes.

6. Allow quesadillas to cool, then cut into fourths. Transfer to serving plate.

7. Serve with salsa, low-fat sour cream, and/or guacamole, if desired. Enjoy!

Yield: 8 servings

## NUTRITION INFORMATION

Serving size: 2 portions

Per serving: 130 calories, 6 g total fat, 2.5 g saturated fat, 15 mg cholesterol, 13 g carbohydrates, 1 g fiber, 2 g sugar, and 160 mg sodium

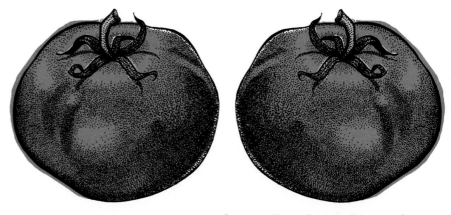

# Green & Orange Pasta Salad

Estimated preparation and cooking time: 20 to 25 minutes, plus an optional
30 minutes of refrigerator time to cool

## INGREDIENTS

1 pound green beans

6 carrots

1 pound whole wheat pasta

2 tablespoons balsamic vinegar

3 tablespoons olive oil

1 cup shredded Parmesan cheese

Salt and pepper to taste

## PROCEDURE

1. Bring pot of water to boil for pasta.

2. Wash green beans and snap off stems.

3. Cut or break green beans into bite-sized pieces and place in steamer or skillet filled with 1½ inches water.

4. Steam or cook green beans over high heat 5–8 minutes or until tender. Cool beans by rinsing under cold water.

5. Wash and peel carrots.

6. Shred carrots in food processor or dice them.

7. When water is boiling, add pasta and cook for 10 minutes or until al dente. When pasta is done, drain in colander. Rinse colander of pasta under cold water.

8. In large bowl, combine vinegar, oil, cheese, salt, and pepper. Add pasta, carrots, and green beans. Mix until combined.

9. Serve immediately or store in refrigerator 30 minutes to cool.

Yield: 12 servings

## NUTRITION INFORMATION

Serving size: $1/12$ recipe

Per serving: 220 calories, 6 g total fat, 2 g saturated fat, 5 mg cholesterol, 35 g carbohydrates, 5 g fiber, 3 g sugar, and 150 mg sodium

# Bell Pepper & Pineapple Fried Rice

Estimated preparation and cooking time: 25 minutes, plus time to cook the rice

## INGREDIENTS

1⅓ cups brown or basmati rice

2 fresh bell peppers, washed

1-inch piece fresh ginger root
(about 2 teaspoons grated)

2 cloves fresh garlic (to yield
about 1 teaspoon crushed)

¼ cup vegetable oil

½ cup canned crushed pineapple
(in its own juice)

2 tablespoons low-sodium, wheat-
free tamari

## PROCEDURE

1. Rinse rice under running water in strainer and place in pot with 2⅔ cups water.

2. Bring to boil. Then lower heat and simmer, covered, 25 minutes or until all water is absorbed and rice is tender. You may need to add a little more water.

3. Remove pot from stove and let sit, covered, 5 minutes.

4. Wash, deseed, and finely chop bell pepper.

5. Peel and finely grate ginger using a cheese grater, or finely dice it.

6. Remove outer skin from garlic cloves, crush cloves in garlic press, or finely chop them.

7. Add to skillet or wok: oil, bell pepper, ginger, and garlic. Raise heat to medium-high and sauté until peppers are soft. Add rice and pineapple.

8. Gently stir mixture to disperse oil and flavorings. Add tamari and heat additional 1–2 minutes.

9. Remove from heat, and allow mixture to cool slightly. Transfer to serving platter. Serve family style.

Yield: 8 servings

## NUTRITION INFORMATION

Serving size: ⅛ recipe

Per serving: 193 calories, 8 g total fat, 1 g saturated fat, 0 mg cholesterol, 28 g carbohydrates, 2 g fiber, 3 g sugar, and 250 mg sodium

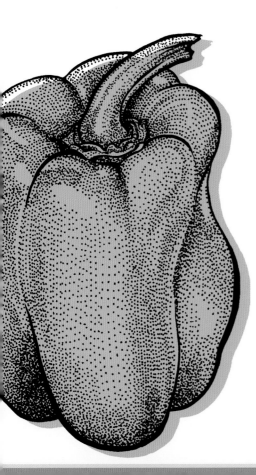

# Butternut Squash Fries

Estimated preparation and cooking time: 50 minutes

## INGREDIENTS

1 medium butternut squash

Salt

Nonstick cooking spray

## PROCEDURE

1. Preheat oven to 425°F. Fill baking dish with about an inch of water.

2. Cut butternut squash in half from top to bottom. Do not scoop out seeds. Place squash cut side down in baking dish with water and bake 20–25 minutes, frequently checking for tenderness. Do not overcook squash.

3. Allow squash to cool thoroughly. Scoop seeds out of squash and discard. Scoop out squash in large chunks.

4. Cut baked squash chunks into french fry shapes.

5. Spray baking sheet with nonstick cooking spray.

6. Place fries on baking sheet. Sprinkle lightly with salt.

7. Place tray in oven and bake 20 minutes, turning fries over halfway through baking process. Fries are done when they start to brown on the edges and get crispy.

8. Serve alone or with favorite condiment or dip.

Yield: 12 servings

## NUTRITION INFORMATION

Serving size: $1/12$ recipe

Per serving: 64 calories, 0 g total fat, 0 g saturated fat, 0 mg cholesterol, 17 g carbohydrates, 3 g fiber, 3 g sugar, and 151 mg sodium

# TEN

~~~

# Partnerships
# with
# Families

The prevalence of obesity in young children is currently rising in the United States. Additionally, more than 11 million children under age five are in some type of child care arrangement every week (NACCRRA 2010). These two facts highlight the importance of child care providers partnering with families to improve the health and nutrition practices of young children. The Early Sprouts approach acknowledges that this partnership is critical and seeks to foster it in a variety of ways.

Early childhood educators understand the importance of relationships with children. Teachers build practices to ensure that children feel safe and secure in child care settings. The National Association for the Education of Young Children (NAEYC) acknowledges the development of this work with standards that address the social and emotional growth and development of young children. Teachers work to create environments that are comfortable, engaging, and developmentally appropriate. In chapter 3, we looked at how early childhood teachers incorporate developmental domains into their curriculum. It is clear that health and nutrition goals are part of the work that teachers do every day. NAEYC accreditation standards include health and nutrition standards and reinforce the commitment of early childhood educators to the healthy growth and development of young children.

While child care providers are usually very comfortable in their work with children, they are less so in dealing with children's families. Developing positive, trusting relationships with families is thoughtful and caring work. "Building relationships with children is different than building relationships with adults" (Keyser 2006, 3). Early childhood educators struggle with building adult relationships, and this includes building relationships that involve food and healthy nutrition practices.

## CREATING A NUTRITIONALLY PURPOSEFUL ENVIRONMENT

It is important for all of us as early childhood professionals to explore our own food histories and begin this journey to a more healthful eating lifestyle with open minds. Changing food habits can be difficult and is often emotionally charged. You may need to examine your own food issues as you begin to explore food issues with families. Did you grow up eating healthy foods? How do you make decisions about what you and your family eat each day? Economic and cultural issues influence our food choices. What are the time pressures you experience, and how do they affect your nutrition decisions? As each of us looks at our own experiences, we can grow in our understanding of others, and the communication between us and families can become more open and constructive.

Begin by assessing the current nutrition and health practices in your program. Collect information by taking a look at your program's responsibilities for providing food. Review your current menus.

- Do you serve one or two snacks per day?

- Do you prepare lunch, or do families provide lunches for children?

- If families provide lunches, are those meals in agreement with CACFP standards and NAEYC accreditation standards?

- How do children and adults respond to the foods served?

- Are families involved in the food program?

- What types of foods are consumed at staff events and potluck dinners with families?

- What do celebrations in your program look like?

Next, explore your thoughts and ideas about nutrition and engage in discussions with other staff members, including teachers, administrators, and support staff. Gather information from the families in your program. You may need to increase staff development and education to ensure that all staff members and families have the information needed to make informed decisions about nutrition and health.

Now you can begin to develop some goals. What is your vision of a nutritionally purposeful environment? Review your assessment information and the attitudes and values of staff, and integrate those with a firm knowledge of nutrition and best practice. The Early Sprouts approach is grounded in nutrition information and child development theory. Within this approach, specific strategies have been identified to positively influence the growth of healthy nutrition practices with young children. These strategies, discussed in chapter 2, include:

- sensory exploration

- multiple exposures

- engaging children in cooking

- family-style meals

- intentional language used with food

- providing only healthy choices

- using teachers and families as role models

The Early Sprouts approach has found that these strategies are highly successful when used in early childhood settings.

Finally, create a plan for change. Changing behaviors is not easy. It takes time and patience. As you begin to make changes in your nutrition environment, remember to provide opportunities for children and adults to explore vegetables and fruit through their senses. With multiple exposures, we all learn more about healthy foods, and we become more comfortable eating them. Cooking in the classroom builds our knowledge of healthy ingredients, engages us in a pleasurable activity, and creates delicious food for us to eat. The Early Sprouts approach also seeks to strengthen the bond between school and home. In *The Cooking Book*, Laura J. Colker states, "Teachers can involve families with cooking in various ways, but inspiring parents to include their children in home cooking activities will have the most lasting effect" (Colker 2005, 49). One of the goals of the Early Sprouts approach is to have long-lasting effects on families: cooking with their children and eating healthy foods.

As you build a plan to create change, you should share the value of that change. Members of your community must embrace the principles of healthy practices. There are many ways to communicate the values of life-long healthy practices. Some of those are listed in the next section, where we explore communication with families. It is important to trust the process as this journey begins. Just as multiple exposures to healthy foods builds children's comfort level with the foods, so multiple exposures to information about healthy practices builds the foundation for adults to make changes in their own practices.

A critical component of the Early Sprouts approach is the role of adults in building nutritionally purposeful environments. Adults have the responsibility to provide healthy choices for children, to engage in family-style meals with children, and to be intentional in their language. Adults are also role models. Children will be more willing to try a new food if adults are trying it with them.

## FAMILY ENGAGEMENT

Traditionally, early childhood educators have viewed the role of working with parents as parent education. The focus has been on providing families with information about parenting in a one-way communication. This practice evolved into parent involvement. The focus of parent involvement has been on teacher- and program-directed activities. The communication between educators and families began to open up, but families were not yet acknowledged for their importance and the strengths they bring in parenting their children. Current practice in the field of early childhood education focuses on family engagement and family-centered care. Developmentally appropriate practice (DAP) clearly articulates NAEYC's position about partnerships between child care providers and families: "Parents are the most important people in their child's life. They know their child well, and their preferences and choices matter. Excellent teachers work hard to develop reciprocal relationships with families, with communication and respect in both directions" (Copple and Bredekamp 2009, 45). The NAEYC accreditation standards (2006) also include the importance of building positive partnerships with families.

> NAEYC Standard 1.A: Building positive relationships among teachers and families
>
> 1.A.01 Teachers work in partnership with families, establishing and maintaining regular, ongoing, two-way communication.
>
> 1.A.05 Teachers share information with families about classroom rules, expectations, and routines not only at enrollment but also as needed throughout the year.

The Early Sprouts approach acknowledges the importance of family relationships in child care environments and shares healthy nutrition practices in a supportive manner.

As a child care provider, you should begin by providing a welcoming environment for families and children. The Early Sprouts approach strives to create a relaxed and positive relationship to healthy foods, cooking, and food-based experiences for children and families. At the same time, you need to clearly communicate expectations and responsibilities. Opportunities for this communication can include interactions with families on the first visit and orientation, the parent handbook, program communication practices, committee involvement, and participation in classroom activities.

## FIRST VISIT AND ORIENTATION

This is the beginning of developing your partnership with families, and it is a critical time for listening and sharing. The Early Sprouts approach is built on a positive and accepting attitude. This attitude should be integrated into the fabric of the program. At the orientation and first visit session, families hear about the importance of healthy nutrition and how it is visible in the program in children's cooking activities, gardening opportunities, snack and meal menus, and more. Parents hear about the important role they will play as members of this community.

## PARENT HANDBOOK

Your parent handbook provides families with information about your nutrition policy, snack menu, and clear policies on lunch packing, birthday celebrations, family potluck events, and other food-related matters. This gives families a clear expectation from your program. Having families included in developing the nutrition policy and other food-related policies provides an opportunity to open explorations of cultural and family value issues and creates a true reflection of the partnership.

## COMMUNICATION PRACTICES

Parents know their child well. Sharing children's experiences between home and child care through daily conversations strengthens the family and teacher partnership. The family's knowledge of their child and their nutrition practices are important. Conversations about the challenges of food preferences and eating practices can be emotionally charged, even stressful. Engaging families in conversations about these relevant issues while acknowledging parents' stresses of working and other time commitments gives teachers important information for developing supportive policies and practices. Open communication between parents and teachers is the foundation of partnerships. The Early Sprouts approach includes daily conversations at drop-off and pickup, the use of notes (from teachers to home and from home to teachers), and newsletters. Health and nutrition are components of all regular parent conferences. Having an open-door policy for families to engage in classroom activities—including food-related activities—supports the flow of communication between teachers and families.

Cooking activities are an integral part of the Early Sprouts approach. When children are cooking regularly in the classroom, they are eager to share their experiences with their families:

- "Mom, I helped to cut the peppers to put in the corn muffins."

- "We used scissors to cut the chard into really small pieces."

- "I was surprised when I cut into the tomato. The seeds splashed out everywhere!"

The Early Sprout approach encourages families to include children in cooking at home. "Anyone who works with young children can attest to the power of partnering with families. Partnership can take many forms in any area of the early childhood program, and cooking is no exception" (Colker 2005, 43). Family life in the twenty-first century is complicated and hectic. Creating relaxed and positive relationships through healthy foods and cooking for children and families can feel like a major challenge, but families find that it has great rewards. Those rewards can extend into grocery shopping adventures and gardening. Since the Early Sprouts program has been implemented in child care programs, early childhood educators are hearing families say things like:

- "Now when we get home, he sits up at the counter in the kitchen and helps me prepare our dinner. We talk and share about our days while we are cooking. I really like it."

- "We are planting our first garden. It really is a great activity for us as a family."

- "Margo is absolutely into the shopping now. She's always gone on shopping trips before, but she would just play with her toys or do whatever she brought with her to amuse herself. Now, especially in the vegetables and fruits, she is very much involved in picking stuff out. She wants to help pick which pepper we're going to bring, which cucumber we're going to bring. And after she got used to doing that in the produce, it's been expanding to the rest of the store as well. She's now an active participant, not just a passenger in the shopping cart, and it did start with the vegetables she was recognizing from Early Sprouts."

## COMMITTEE INVOLVEMENT

Whether you have an existing health and nutrition committee or will be starting a new one, this is an excellent opportunity for families to share their ideas. It stimulates your child care community to create policies that meet its needs and that reflect its culture. It also offers an excellent opportunity to share knowledge about nutrition and how the child care program and families can work together on a nutritious diet and healthy lifestyle. Committee work could also include:

- Developing kits with a recipe and ingredients to send home to encourage families to cook at home with children

- Building community resources for healthy foods—looking into Community Supported Agriculture (CSA) farms and negotiating with them for fresh produce in the growing season

- Planting a garden with children and families

- Organizing family members to come into the classroom to cook with children

- Creating special events, such as a stone soup lunch, a pancake breakfast (featuring whole grains), or a garden party

- Developing nutrition education workshops, including "How to pack a healthy lunch" and "Understanding and using the USDA's MyPlate"

- Creating family cooking events that acknowledge and respect the diversity of the community—for example, Dad's Night Out (dads join their children in cooking activities in the classroom)

- Sponsoring a family pizza party at which families join their children in creating healthy pizzas for dinner

- Participating in classroom activities and classroom documentation

Encouraging families to join in classroom activities, share their talents and interests, and engage in the classroom community helps to build strong bonds among families, children, and teachers. Negotiation can be a part of these interactions to insure that the values you have outlined in your parent handbook are honored. For example, teachers in one Early Sprouts preschool classroom asked families about their interests and the ways they could participate in classroom activities. One parent enthusiastically offered her skills in cake decorating. "I could bring in my pastry tubes with frosting and children could decorate cookies!" The teachers acknowledged her excitement and began to think of a way to include this activity in a way that agreed with a healthy and nutritious environment. After some brainstorming together, the parent and teacher agreed that the parent would use hummus in her pastry tubes and decorate freshly cut vegetables, including carrots and bell pepper strips. The event was a great success! The parent was able to share her passion for cake decorating, and the children were provided with healthy food. It was a creative solution that valued the interest of a family while continuing to support healthy eating.

As parents spend time in the classroom, they see bulletin boards and documentation of children engaged in activities. Early Sprouts classroom teachers can take photos of children engaged in sensory exploration and cooking activities. When these photos are displayed along with children's thoughts and ideas, the joy and learning become more visible to everyone. In one preschool classroom, photos of children participating in a cooking activity included this exchange:

> "I love peppers!" said Nick. Zander responded, "Me too. We ate them all up lickety-split." The teacher said, "I am glad you like the peppers, but please save some for the recipe." Aiden cut into his pepper and was surprised when it splashed onto his face. He said, "Wow, these peppers are really juicy." He popped a piece of pepper in the bowl and one into his mouth. "One for the recipe and one for me!" he exclaimed.

Families who have embraced the program find joy in cooking, grocery shopping, and gardening with their children. When adults share in this sense of wonder with their young children, the parent-child bond grows stronger. We encourage you to help families begin with small changes.

The recipes in this book are simple. Changing eating habits is a learning process for everyone—children, families, and teachers. It is a journey that progresses over time. Persistence is the key. We can all celebrate simple changes, such as regularly including cherry tomatoes in your lunch or adding Swiss chard to your pasta sauce. Once again, it is important for families, teachers, and other adults in children's lives to be open to new possibilities.

. . . . . . . . . . . . . . . .
## CONCLUSION

Karen is the single mom of a four-year-old. On a Thursday afternoon, she came to pick up Tristan at the child care center. She found the first Early Sprouts family recipe kit of the year in his cubby. Michelle, the classroom teacher, enthusiastically greeted her and began sharing more information about the Early Sprouts program. Karen looked at the teacher and sighed. "He won't eat this. He hates vegetables. I have tried everything. I beg and plead. I tried explaining the importance of eating healthy foods. I have tried to hide vegetables in his food. That didn't work. I get so frustrated that sometimes I yell, sometimes I cry. I just don't know what to do. I want to be a good parent. I want him to eat healthy food, but . . . I just don't know what to do."

Michelle listened to Karen and heard her concerns. Karen is a caring parent who loves her child. She has many stresses in her life, commuting from home to child care to work. She is struggling to be what she sees as a good parent, and she finds it difficult. We can all empathize with her challenges. Early childhood teachers must begin at the beginning and continue with conversations throughout the year. In that moment, Michelle empathized with Karen's struggle and encouraged her to be patient. Building healthy eating practices can take time. She reassured Karen that they would be together on this journey.

As time passed, Tristan began joining in classroom exploration and cooking activities. Michelle shared Tristan's experiences in the classroom with his mom on a regular basis. She continued to support him with "I understand that you don't like this yet" as he continued to say that he didn't eat vegetables. Then one week, as he was preparing a recipe with other children, he tasted the bell peppers. When his mom came to pick him up, he happily grabbed his family recipe kit and said, "Mom, I really like this one!"

This journey to creating a nutritionally purposeful environment in our child care programs and in our partnerships with families can be challenging but also joyful. The look of surprise on a child's face the first time he cuts open a bell pepper, and the smile that comes when a child picks a cherry tomato off the garden vine, pops it in her mouth and discovers the sweet juicy taste are extraordinarily rewarding. The excitement in parents' voices when they share the process of planting their family garden or realize that they do like the taste of butternut squash pancakes is a positive step in developing a healthier family environment.

Enjoying whole grains, low-fat dairy, fruits, and vegetables creates a happy, healthy environment for young children to grow in. Cooking and eating together as a family builds positive relationships. The Early Sprouts approach incorporates early childhood theory and practice, and nutrition research to provide a nutritionally purposeful child care environment.

# APPENDIX

## CHILDREN'S PICTURE BOOK LIST

*Bread, Bread, Bread* by Ann Morris. Lothrop, Lee & Shepard, 1989.
> Bread can come in many forms. As a bagel, a tortilla, or a baguette, bread is eaten by people all around the world. Accompanying the simple text are vibrant color photographs of kinds of bread baked in different countries around the world.

*The Carrot Seed* by Ruth Krauss. Harper & Row, 1945.
> A little boy plants a carrot seed and patiently tends to it despite those around him insisting, "It won't come up." The boy's faith and determination are rewarded with a carrot so large that it wins first prize at the state fair. Young readers learn the value of dedication and standing one's ground.

*Chop, Simmer, Season* by Alexa Brandenberg. Harcourt, 1997.
> A man and woman cook a meal for awaiting customers at the Top Notch Restaurant. The text, all verbs, such as "peel," "sauté," and "mash," are accompanied by close up illustrations of food preparation. Although the order may seem random, the verbs are placed in a specific order as the two chefs prepare a specific meal.

*Eating the Alphabet* by Lois Ehlert. Harcourt Brace Jovanovich, 1989.
> This appetizing alphabet book illustrates fruits and veggies from "Apple to Zucchini" with mouthwatering watercolor collages. Easy to read, this book also includes a glossary that provides pronunciation, origin and history, botanical information, and the occasional mythological reference that children will enjoy.

*The Enormous Carrot* by Vladimir Vagin. Scholastic, 1998.
> A variation of "The Enormous Turnip," this story features two rabbits who find a large carrot but cannot pull it out of the ground even with the help of their barnyard neighbors. Only when Lester the Mouse joins the group can they free it from the soil. The story concludes with carrot-themed feast of cakes, cookies, soup and more, and a learned lesson of cooperation.

*Feast for 10* by Cathryn Falwell. Clarion, 1993.
> Readers count from one to ten twice as an African American family goes shopping for and then prepares a feast for their extended family ("ten hungry folks"). The rhyme scheme and colorful cut-paper illustrations create homey, family-centered images.

*Grandpa's Garden Lunch* by Judith Casely. Greenwillow, 1990.
> This story focuses on Sarah and her grandfather as they plant and tend to vegetables, flowers, and herbs, all illustrated in bright watercolors. After they finish, Sarah and her grandparents enjoy the fruits of their labor.

*Growing Vegetable Soup* by Lois Ehlert. Harcourt Brace Jovanovich, 1987.
> This book features vivid abstract artwork that illustrates the complete growing process— from planting seeds and watering them to harvesting the vegetables and cooking them. This fresh presentation is accompanied by an easy recipe for vegetable soup.

*The Little Red Hen (Makes a Pizza)* by Philemon Sturges. Dutton Children's Books, 1999.
When Hen decides to make a pizza, her neighbors seem disinterested. But when she buys the ingredients at the store (and a few unnecessary items) and bakes the pizza, her neighbors quickly change their tune. This zany retelling of the Little Red Hen is perfectly partnered with wacky cut-paper images.

*Lunch* by Denise Fleming. Henry Holt and Co, 1992.
A mouse nibbles his way through a feast of colorful and tasty fruits and vegetables, enhanced by vibrant illustrations that practically drench the page.

*One Bean* by Anne Rockwell. Walker and Co, 1998.
A young narrator describes how a bean grows from a simple wet paper towel to the full-fledged plant bearing beans of its own bean pods. An introduction to plant growth and observation, this book also includes activities children can do themselves.

*Pancakes, Pancakes* by Eric Carle. Simon & Schuster, 1990.
Featuring Carle's familiar, colorful collages, Jack decides he wants pancakes for breakfast. But his mother must first collect all the ingredients from the mill, a chicken, and a cow before she can begin making the pancake of Jack's dreams.

*Red Are the Apples* by Marc Harshman and Cheryl Ryan. Gulliver Books, 2001.
A boy and some farm animals wander through a farm's abundant fields and inspect the apples, pumpkins, lima beans, eggplants, corn, and beets, which are with pastels befitting of autumn.

*Stone Soup* by Jon Muth. Scholastic, 2003.
Muth transports this familiar folktale to China, where three Zen monks arrive in an unwelcoming village full of selfish residents. By brewing stone soup and drawing villagers forth to add ingredients, the monks teach the village the value of sharing.

*This Is the Bread I Baked for Ned* by Crescent Dragonwagon. Athenium, 1989.
In cumulative verse, the narrator describes how she first bakes bread for Ned, and then cheese and salad and soup and more. But when Ned brings home thirteen guests, will there be enough food to go around?

*Today Is Monday* by Eric Carle. Philomel Books, 1993.
This book captures the well-known children's song with an array of boldly colorful animals who feast on their favorite foods. The final spread depicts a grand banquet enjoyed by multiethnic children while the animals watch from paintings on the wall.

*Up, Down, and Around* by Kathrine Ayres. Candlewick Press, 2007.
This upbeat story introduces children to gardening and prepositions through the use of rhyme. Two children learn—as noted in the title—plants can grow up out of the ground, down underground, and on vines that coil around and around.

*The Vegetables We Eat* by Gail Gibbons. Holiday House, 2007.
Featuring bright watercolor-and-ink artwork and fun facts, this book is an inviting introduction to vegetables. The book shows both small- and large-scale production through scenes in a garden, on a farm, and at a supermarket.

# REFERENCES

Berman, Christine, and Jacki Fromer. 2006. *Meals without Squeals: Child Care Feeding Guide and Cookbook.* Boulder, CO: Bull Publishing Company.

Birch, Leann Lipps, and Jennifer A. Fisher. 1996. "The Role of Experience in the Development of Children's Eating Behavior." In *Why We Eat What We Eat: The Psychology of Eating*, edited by Elizabeth D. Capaldi, 113–41. Washington, DC: American Psychological Association.

Birch, Leann Lipps, and Diane Wolfe Marlin. 1982. "I Don't Like It; I Never Tried It: Effects of Exposure on Two-Year-Old Children's Food Preferences." *Appetite* 3 (4): 353–60.

Cadwell, Louise Boyd. 1997. *Bringing Reggio Emilia Home: An Innovative Approach to Early Childhood Education.* New York: Teachers College Press.

Carson, Rachel. 1998. *The Sense of Wonder.* New York: HarperCollins.

Colker, Laura J. 2005. *The Cooking Book: Fostering Young Children's Learning and Delight.* Washington, DC: National Association for the Education of Young Children.

Copple, Carol, and Sue Bredekamp, eds. 2009. *Developmentally Appropriate Practice in Early Childhood Programs.* 3rd ed. Washington, DC: National Association for the Education of Young Children.

Dodge, Diane Trister, Laura J. Colker, and Cate Heroman. 2002. *The Creative Curriculum for Preschool.* 4th ed. Washington, DC: Teaching Strategies.

Fungwe, Thomas, Patricia M. Guenther, WenYen Juan, Hazel Hiza, and Mark Lino. 2009. "The Quality of Children's Diets in 2003–04 as Measured by the Healthy Eating Index–2005." United States Department of Agriculture. www.cnpp.usda.gov/Publications/NutritionInsights/Insight43.pdf.

Gallo, Anthony E. 1999. "Food Advertising in the United States." In *America's Eating Habits: Changes and Consequences*, edited by Elizabeth Frazao, 173–80. United States Department of Agriculture. Washington, DC: United States Government Printing Office.

Hessert, Bill. 2005. "New Research Center to Tackle Childhood Obesity Epidemic." *Penn State Live.* live.psu.edu/story/13259.

Johnson, Rachel K., Lawrence J. Appel, Michael Brands, Barbara V. Howard, Michael Lefevre, Robert H. Lustig, Frank Sacks, Lyn M. Steffen, and Judith Wyle-Rosett. 2009. "Dietary Sugars Intake and Cardiovascular Health: A Scientific Statement from the American Heart Association." *Circulation* 120: 1011–20. doi:10.1161/circulationaha.109.192627.

Johnson, Susan L., and Leann Lipps Birch. 1994. "Parents' and Children's Adiposity and Eating Style." *Pediatrics* 94 (5): 653–61.

Jones, Elizabeth, and John Nimmo. 1994. *Emergent Curriculum.* Washington, DC: National Association for the Education of Young Children.

Katz, Lilian G., and Sylvia C. Chard. 2000. *Engaging Children's Minds: The Project Approach.* Stamford, CT: Ablex Publishing.

Keyser, Janis. 2006. *From Parents to Partners: Building a Family-Centered Early Childhood Program.* St. Paul, MN: Redleaf Press.

NAEYC (National Association for the Education of Young Children). 2005. *Early Childhood Program Standards and Accreditation Criteria.* Washington, DC: National Association for the Education of Young Children.

———. 2006. *Guidance on NAEYC Accreditation Criteria.* Washington, DC: National Association for the Education of Young Children.

———. 2009. *Developmentally Appropriate Practice in Early Childhood Programs Serving Children from Birth through Age 8: A Position Statement of the National Association for the Education of Young Children.* Washington, DC: National Association for the Education of Young Children.

NAEYC (National Association for the Education of Young Children) and the National Association of Early Childhood Specialists in the State Department of Education (NAECS/SDE). 2002. *Early Learning Standards: Creating the Conditions for Success.* A joint position statement of the National Association for the Education of Young Children (NAEYC) and the National Association of Early Childhood Specialists in the State Department of Education (NAECS/SDE). www.naeyc.org/files/naeyc/file/positions/executive_summary.pdf.

National Association of Child Care Resource and Referral Agencies (NACCRRA). 2010. *The Economy's Impact on Parents' Choices and Perceptions about Child Care.*

National Cancer Institute. 2010. "Usual Intake of Added Sugars." From "Usual Dietary Intakes: Food Intakes, US Population, 2001–04." National Cancer Institute. riskfactor.cancer.gov/diet/usualintakes/pop/added_sugars.html.

Ogden, Cynthia L., Margaret D. Carroll, and Katherine M. Flegal. 2008. "High Body Mass Index for Age Among US Children and Adolescents, 2003–2006." *JAMA* 299 (20): 2401–5. doi:10.1001/jama.299.20.2401.

Satter, E. 2000. *Child of Mine: Feeding with Love and Good Sense.* Boulder, CO: Bull Publishing Company.

Sullivan, Susan A., and Leann Lipps Birch. 1994. "Infant Dietary Experience and Acceptance of Solid Foods." *Pediatrics* 93 (2): 271–77.

United States Department of Agriculture and United States Department of Health and Human Services. 2010. *Dietary Guidelines for Americans, 2010.* Washington, DC: United States Government Printing Office.

United States Department of Health and Human Services. 2010. *The Head Start Child Development and Early Learning Framework.* Arlington, VA.

# SUBJECT INDEX

## A

adult-child conversations during mealtimes, 37

adult diseases and conditions in children and adolescents, 2

adults
and children's poor dietary choices, 19
role in Early Sprouts approach, 169–172
as role models, 38

advertising, and eating habits, 1

antioxidants, 6

appliances, small, 42

assessment practices, 30, 170

## B

behavior change, 168–169, 175, 178

birthday celebrations, 25
*See also* Recipes Index

bran, in processed grains, 7

breakfast, CACFP requirements for, 47

breakfast recipes. *See* Recipes Index

## C

CACFP. *See* Child and Adult Care Food Program (CACFP)

calcium, in dairy-based and nondairy foods, 8

Carson, Rachel, 32

celebrations, 125
*See also* Recipes Index

cereal, sugar content, 9

Child and Adult Care Food Program (CACFP)
breakfast components required, 47
in healthy eating for preschool children, 13–14
lunch components required, 71
snack components required, 95

child care centers, CACFP and, 13–14

cleaning materials, 44–45

cleanup, 44–45

cognitive development, 32–33

cola soft drinks, sugar content, 9

Colker, Laura J., 37

committee involvement, in family engagement, 172–174

communication and language development, 35–36

communication practices, in family engagement, 170–172

cooking environments, child-friendly, 41–44

cooking with young children, 41–46
benefits, 21–22
cause-and-effect learning, 33
cooperation in, 37, 43–44
families and, 173
and physical development in young children, 22, 34–35
safety in, 42–44
and social-emotional development, 37–38
tools for, 42

cooperation, in cooking, 37, 43–44

cracking eggs, 37–38

## D

dairy, in healthy eating, 8–9

dairy-free alternatives, 8

DAP. *See* developmentally appropriate practice (DAP)

Department of Health and Human Services Administration for Children and Families, 30

developmentally appropriate practice (DAP)
defined, 27–28
early childhood educators and, 30
Early Sprouts approach, 31, 39
kitchen tasks, 35

dietary fiber, 8, 63

dietary needs for preschool-age children, 3–4

## E

early childhood educators
developmentally appropriate practices and, 30
dietary habits of, 168–169
as role models, 19, 22, 24–25, 38, 71

early childhood nutrition, 1–14

Early Learning Guidelines (ELGs), 28–32, 36–38, 39

Early Sprouts approach
basis of, 16
DAP in, 31
to family engagement, 170–174
food philosophy, 25
goals of, 1
meaning of, 15–16
nutritional philosophy in, 17–20
role of adults in, 169–170
sensory exploration in, 20–21
starting early, 16–17

eggs
cracking, 37–38
in healthy eating for preschool children, 9

ELGs (Early Learning Guidelines), 28–32, 36–38, 39

emergent curricula, and Early Sprouts approach, 31

## F

family-centered care, 170

family engagement
building relationships, 167
committee involvement, 172–174
communication practices, 171–172
creating nutritionally purposeful environments, 168–170
Early Sprouts approach to, 170–174
intentional language about food, 23
as role models, 19, 24, 25

family mealtime, avoiding conflict, 23–24

family recipe kits, 173

family-style meals, 22–23, 38

fats, healthy, 9–10

fatty acids, 10

fiber, 8, 63

fish, in healthy eating, 9–10

flour, enriched, 7

Food Guide Pyramid, USDA, 2–3

# RECIPES AND INGREDIENTS INDEX

Note: Boldface type indicates recipe titles as they appear in the cookbook.

# Cultivate healthy change in your classroom and plant the seeds for healthy eating habits.

If you like the recipes in *The Early Sprouts Cookbook,* check out the nutrition and gardening curriculum that started it all!

*Early Sprouts* helps children choose to eat and grow healthy foods and includes

- Guidelines for establishing garden beds

- Strategies for sensory explorations that enhance children's scientific and literacy development and provide knowledge about vegetables

- Healthy recipes specifically designed to be used with young children

- Tips for involving teachers and families in improving everyone's personal eating habits

## Early Sprouts

Cultivating Healthy Food Choices in Young Children

**Karrie Kalich, Dottie Bauer, and Deirdre McPartlin**

AWARD Winner

The *Early Sprouts* program received the Community Champion Award from the U.S. Surgeon General for its "commitment to building partnerships and implementing programs to help kids stay active, encourage kids' healthy eating habits, and promote healthy choices."

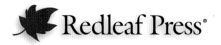 Redleaf Press®